YOU▮
IS DI▮

A handbook for ▮▮▮▮▮ ▮▮▮▮▮ ▮▮▮▮▮▮
with special needs

EDITED BY DAVID MITCHELL
THIS EDITION ADAPTED
BY JANET HORWOOD

LONDON
UNWIN PAPERBACKS
BOSTON SYDNEY

First published in Great Britain by Unwin
Paperbacks 1982

UNWIN® PAPERBACKS
40 Museum Street, London, WC1A 1LU, UK

Unwin Paperbacks
Park Lane, Hemel Hempstead, Herts HP2 4TE,
UK

©David Mitchell 1982
UK additions © George Allen & Unwin
(Publishers) Ltd 1982

ISBN 0 04 649016 7

Set in 10/11 pt English Times
Colset Pte Ltd, Singapore
Printed by Bright Sun Printing Press Co., Ltd. Hong Kong

Contents

1 To Put You in the Picture

Background

We have written this book mainly for parents of young handicapped children, but we hope that it will also be of benefit to professional workers. We also hope that it will be helpful to *all* parents of young children. Although handicapped children pose some special challenges, a great deal of what we recommend to help their development is relevant to all children.

The book was originally written to accompany a series of broadcasts produced by the Continuing Education Unit of Radio New Zealand to mark the 1979 International Year of the Child. The material in this book has been prepared by several people, most of whom are associated with two New Zealand projects aimed at helping parents of young children with special needs – Dawnstart Project in Wellington and Project PATH in Hamilton. Since our backgrounds are mainly in the fields of psychology, teaching, and speech therapy, we have largely confined ourselves to these areas. We haven't gone into medical matters; if you have any concerns about your child's health, you should discuss these with your family doctor or your paediatrician.

The Focus of this Book

Throughout this book we will be referring to children with special needs. Although our concern is with the whole range, most of our examples will be drawn from children whose special needs are intellectual and physical. We make only occasional references to children with vision or hearing handicaps.

Does Your Child Have Special Needs?

All parents think of their own children as quite unique. This is true, of course, for children differ not only in their appearance, but also in the way they move, the way they relate to others, the way they process information, the way they express themselves in words and gestures . . . For the most part, these differences are quite acceptable – even desirable, for who wants all children to be the same! But, in about one in ten children these differences cause concern. Those are the children who have more difficulty than most in learning or in controlling their movements, who have visual or hearing disabilities, or major behaviour problems. They are children who are different in a special kind of way and sometimes very difficult to manage.

Your child might already have been professionally diagnosed as having an intellectual handicap or a physical handicap, or as being deaf or blind. It may be, however, that at this stage you merely suspect that your child has special needs.

The following checklist might help you to decide if it is worth discussing your child with somebody professionally qualified to assess and advise on children's development – and whether this book is specially relevant to you.

Since there is a great deal of variability among normal children, however, you should not become too concerned unless your child is extremely delayed or has difficulties in several areas.

☐ has not held head erect by 5 months
☐ has not rolled over by 7 months
☐ has not sat unsupported by 11 months
☐ has not begun to feed himself by 12 months
☐ has not said first word by 15 months
☐ has not walked unsupported by 18 months

☐ has not drunk unassisted from a cup by 24 months
☐ has not put 2 or 3 words together in a simple sentence by 24 months
☐ has not copied your drawing of a circle by 30 months
☐ has not achieved daytime bladder control by 30 months
☐ has difficulty in controlling hand movements
☐ does not respond to sounds, especially if their sources can't be seen
☐ prefers to sit very close to the television
☐ frequently rubs his eyes
☐ does not relate to other people and may even resist them
☐ is unusually active or passive
☐ is very aggressive towards other children
☐ has a marked stammer
☐ persistently engages in behaviour such as head banging and rocking
☐ is unusually clumsy

(*Note*: the ages in this checklist refer to the ages by which almost all children have achieved the items.)

He/She

We are aware of the problems of writing about babies and children without suggesting they are all boys (by referring to 'him' all the time). We also wanted to avoid clumsy constructions such as 'he/she', or cold terms like 'it'. Our solution has been to use 'he' for some sections and 'she' for others. We hope you like our compromise.

Underlying Ideas

Most sections of this book will give you practical suggestions on ways you can help your child develop. Before you read these, however, you might like to know some of the ideas which underlie our suggestions:

The Family as Teachers

In the first place, we firmly believe that *the family plays a very important part* in helping children with special needs. This is especially true in the first few years when you, his parents, are your child's main teachers. You see more of him and probably know more about him and his abilities than anyone else. We feel, too, that his brothers and sisters and his grandparents play an important role, right from these early years.

Early Experiences Count

Our second underlying idea is that *early experiences are very important*. While it is true that it's almost never too late to learn some things, there are many skills which are more readily learned in the first few years. In the early years, all children require stimulating as well as loving experiences with people – especially their family. Teaching and learning begins well before they go to preschool, school, or a special care centre. You can help your child's development right from birth.

Have Realistic Expectations

The third point we would like to make is that, if given proper stimulation and training, children with special needs are *capable of far more than was once thought possible*. The old idea that they just needed to be looked after or kept occupied has gone. Now they are being helped to live as normally and as independently as possible within the community. Of course, there will be limits to what your child can achieve, but these limits are generally much higher than was thought twenty, ten and even five years ago. This means that you as a parent must work out realistic expectations for *your* child – not too high and certainly not too low. Your child is an individual first and foremost, so get to know his strengths and weaknesses. A father of a Down's Syndrome boy nicely summed up this point: 'I think you've got to have some motivation in it, something in which the child is trying to push himself a bit further forward. It's no use giving him something he can do.'

A similar attitude was expressed by the mother of a severely handicapped child: 'As long as you don't expect a miracle, as long as you don't expect them to do greater and better things, because that is when you can be very disappointed. But so long as you don't just give up trying with them . . .'

Seek Professional Help

While most of our activities can be managed without the direct assistance of a professional person, it is much better that *you talk them over with someone who knows* about children with special needs. It may be, for example, that your child's environment needs to be arranged so that he can make the most of it or that he needs special furniture and equipment. As a mother of a cerebral palsied boy expressed it, 'If I'd known what to ask for – you don't know what's available. You find out months later you could or should have had something – a piece of equipment, home aid, or ideas about how to help your child to do something you thought he'd find impossible because of his handicap.'

Your family doctor and paediatrician are possible sources of help, but here is a list of others who can assist you. You can contact them directly yourself; or through your doctor or paediatrician; Health or Education Department Psychologists.

- ☐ child guidance counsellors
- ☐ speech therapists
- ☐ teachers in special schools
- ☐ community nurses or social workers
- ☐ social workers and advisers with voluntary societies
- ☐ parent groups

While you may not always have ready access to all of these people, try to consult those who might be able to offer you relevant advice. A list of services available to families of children with special needs is included in a section at the end of this book.

Keep a Balance

So far we have emphasized the important part that your family can play in helping your child to develop. You may now be wondering just how much you could reasonably be expected to do to help him. Obviously, this will vary from child to child, depending upon the extent of his problems. Our fifth guiding principle, however, is that it is *important to keep a balance* – a point that underlies our answers to some questions you may be asking:

Will we need lots of expensive equipment?
No. Most of the activities we recommend are simple, everyday things most parents do with their children. Most of them can, and should, become part of playing with your child.

Will we need lots of extra assistance?
No. You won't need to get help from large numbers of friends or relatives to carry out the activities. We do hope, however, that everyone in your family will become involved in some way and as regularly as possible.

Do we need to spend a lot of time with him?
This depends on many things: the extent of your child's special needs, whether or not you are working on a supervised programme with him, your own commitments . . . . Our feeling is that the important thing is not so much *how long* you should spend with your child, but *how well* you use the time you do spend with him.

By and large, most of the activities in this book can be included in your everyday routine. However, you might like to set aside a few minutes 'special time' each day to concentrate on certain skills. Try to make sure these times are least likely to be interrupted by your other children, neighbours popping in, pots boiling over . . . . Choose times when your child is most likely to be alert and interested in what's going on.

Look, too, for ways of making them happy times. Especially, try to begin and end each session with something you both enjoy.

Just how important is our child with special needs?
Very important, but not so important that you neglect other members of the family – your husband, your wife, your other children, yourself . . . . Don't feel guilty if you want to take a break. Your child needs a strong, happy parent and you owe that to yourself anyway! Don't forget that, as the mother of a deaf girl said, 'The other children in the family need to feel they are important. It is very distressing when they have to be pushed into the background. This really worries me!'

Children with Special Needs have Rights

In the last ten years or so, society's attitudes towards children with special needs have changed considerably, and for the better. There is now much more understanding of their needs and those of their families. We think this change in attitude reflects several things that are taking place.

Firstly, there is the vast increase in research and publishing about children with special needs, much of this reflecting *optimism* about their potential to develop skills if the right conditions are provided.

Secondly, there is the air of *hope and determination* that has been generated by you, the parents of children with special needs. Sometimes this has been accomplished through the efforts of individual parents demonstrating to their friends, relatives and neighbours that such children can lead satisfying and full lives. Sometimes it has been brought about by the public relations efforts of the voluntary societies acting on your behalf.

Thirdly, there is the growing recognition in society that children with special needs have *rights*. The United Nations Declaration of Childrens' Rights, for example, contains this principle:
The child who is physically, mentally or socially handicapped shall be given the special treatment, education and care required by his particular condition.
We believe, too, that the United Nations Declaration on the Rights of Mentally Retarded Persons is applicable to all children with special needs:

Whenever possible, the mentally retarded person should live with his own family or with foster parents and participate in different forms of community life. The family with which he lives should receive assistance. If care in an institution becomes necessary, it should be provided in surroundings and other circumstances as close as possible to those of normal life.

Have Confidence in your own Ability

As you read this book and try out the ideas, you will probably be saying, 'But what's new – I did that with my other children?' Or, if you are a new parent you might be saying, 'But this is what I would have been doing even if my child wasn't handicapped'.

By and large, you will be quite right, for children with special needs are not all that different from other children. They learn things in much the same way, even if progress at times seems painfully slow. They have the same needs for love and attention. They will make you angry and they will make you happy . . . .

Although you will have to pay more attention to setting goals for your child and you will have to adjust yourself to a slower pace of learning, *have confidence in your own ability* as a parent. Common sense will get you a long way with helping your child to develop.

Have Fun!

It all sounds rather serious, doesn't it? Certainly, there is a serious side to having a child with special needs in your family, but there is no reason why you can't *have fun and enjoyment* as you go about trying to help him. We really do hope that you will think of the activities we suggest as games rather than as burdensome 'lessons'. Relax and enjoy doing them with your child.

David Mitchell

2 Getting Used to Each Other

The sooner you come to that state of being able to say, 'I have a handicapped child' – to be able to say that without feeling embarrassment, you're THERE!

Mother of severely handicapped child.

All children are a challenge to their parents' ingenuity and patience at times. At other times, they are bringers of great joy and satisfaction. The same is true of children with special needs – but more so. Parents have to make greater efforts with them, but also tell us of the triumphs the family can enjoy when the disabled one achieves a new skill – 'I expected it with my others, but we went over the moon when Sharon learnt to feed herself'. They also tell us of the pleasure they have when their child begins to relate to them as a *person*.

Let's not forget the other side, though. The shock when you first heard the news. The sorrow of watching your child in pain. The anger and frustration you might feel when a longed-for development is slow in coming. The times you say to yourself, 'Why did it happen to me?'

In this chapter, we will look at two aspects of getting used to your child with special needs:

☐ Firstly, we will discuss some of the *difficult feelings* you as parents or as a family of a handicapped child have to cope with. We will give some suggestions about how to change or cope with these feelings, in the hope that, during the bad times especially, you will be able to understand a bit more about why you feel the way you do, and what you can do about it.

☐ Secondly, we will look at the question of *how parents really become parents*. Here, we will focus on the importance of 'bonds' between children and their parents and how these bonds can be created and made stronger.

FEELINGS

We believe it is extremely important for you, as parents of a child with special needs, to give consideration to the way you feel. To cope with your child, to carry out the ideas in this book, you need to feel pretty good about yourself. Your life, your marriage, your work, need to be bringing you a fair amount of satisfaction. You may deep down always be sad about the fact your child is handicapped. But that need not colour your whole life grey. So let's look now at some of these feelings and ways people have found to cope with them.

The feelings we are particularly concerned about are the 'bad' ones – shock, numbness, confusion, anger, bitterness, sorrow, shame, guilt. People usually know how to express good feelings, but are often scared of the bad ones. We often think that we aren't supposed to feel bad. We think, too, that people don't want to know about our problems and will think worse of us if they did. Because of this, and also because nobody wants to feel bad, we push such feelings down and try to carry on as usual. They don't go away though, and the longer they are held down, or repressed, the more they may affect our lives – and the lives of our families, friends and work-mates.

Perhaps the first thing to say is that the way you feel about your child, and the effects on your way of life, *is one of the normal ways people react to situations which demand a lot of them*. There is nothing special or abnormal about your feelings. You might feel a great sense of determination to succeed with your child, or a sickening ache of depression when she wets the floor yet again. Or maybe you have taught yourself not to feel anything; that way life is dull but at least it is less painful. These reactions are all normal. This is how people feel – only we don't often talk about it. And you may talk about it less than some because having a handicapped child can cut you off *if you let it*. You can feel that people don't want to know, or feel too embarrassed to ask about your child. Or your feelings can mean that you don't want to talk about it with outsiders. Either way, it can lead to you keeping your feelings to yourself. Perhaps you don't even share them with your husband or wife. That can be hard on you, so the first thing you should know is this:

You are not strange or wicked because you have strong feelings. They are nothing to be ashamed of.

The second thing is this:

You probably need to talk more about how you are really feeling.

Almost everyone does. It is something we are not helped or encouraged to do, but we really need to do it. Sometimes talking helps us to let off steam, and sometimes it helps us to get to crying. Yes, crying; not just on our own when we get to the end of our tether, but with someone – a relative, a friend or a counsellor – on whose sympathy and understanding we can rely. Crying with someone can be a very healing way of releasing bad feelings. It is not a sign of weakness. It can often be a sign that you have the strength to recognise – and to cope with – your feelings.

The third point to make is that:

Different people react in different ways to the same situation.

Some of this is to do with us, the way we are as individuals. Some of it is due to the way things are, and the amount of support we get.

Let's look back now to the time you were first told that your child was different. Perhaps this was when she was just born, or during her first few months of life. Or perhaps it was not until she failed to walk or talk, after many months of anxious wondering and worrying on your part. How do people typically react to this knowledge? In the rest of this section, we will talk about these reactions and how you might cope with them.

Grief

That first unwelcome news that your child was different may well have started you off on a process like *grieving* for the death of a loved one. In a sense, it is a death. It is the death of your dream of a normal child and the start of your journey towards acceptance and understanding of the child you have got. Some parents take a long time to forget that dream child and, until they do, find it hard to get to know and love their real child.

Shock

For most, if not all, parents, the first reactions are *shock*, which can take the form of numbness, or sobbing, or even appearing not to care. You may have disbelieved what you were hearing, or been confused and unable to take it in. Maybe the news came as no surprise, but even so, caused you to feel very sick inside. Whatever you felt, it probably took you some time to get over it. Perhaps, you are not 'over it' yet. If you have recently had such news, could we suggest you do the following things, if they have not been arranged already?

☐ You may have found it very difficult to take in what you were being told. You may have many questions to ask. You need to be able to talk several times with someone who knows what is wrong with your child and the problems you may face. You also need to know where you can get the medical, social and educational help your child will need in her early years.

☐ If you are having trouble getting the message across to your relatives, especially the child's grandparents, you might like to ask the person who has been helping you to talk to them too.
In chapter 10, we list some of the people and services who can help you at this time.

☐ During this shock stage, you may find it hard to do what you have to do at home and at work. Don't worry, you aren't losing your grip. This is part of your own safety mechanism. In order to cope with the shock, your body wants you to slow down and make things as easy as possible for yourself. If you can get somebody to stay and help you in the house, so much the better. If you can get time off work, or reduce your work-load, do it. This is a temporary phase. You will soon be able to cope again, so long as you *give yourself time* to get over the shock.

Disbelief and Protest

You just can't believe he is your child when you are first told.

Mother of spina bifida boy.

For most parents, the stage of shock is followed by one of *disbelief* and *protest*. Because the facts are so unacceptable, you may try to deny them and look for hope elsewhere. Perhaps next time the doctor sees your child, he will say he is wrong. Perhaps another specialist will know better, will have a cure . . . . It is a very natural feeling to wish that problems were not there – and from that point, to go one step further and say they do not exist at all. Sometimes parents deny that their child has a problem and will not accept the help that is offered. Or they may accept that their child is different, but believe that some miracle will cure her – new drugs, an operation, a programme of exercises taking many hours each day. Or maybe they think if they just love her enough, she will get well. Sometimes, you may hope so much for things to be all right that you wish your child would die. As a mother of a Down's Syndrome girl said, 'Especially just after she was born, I kept on thinking "I wish she would die" . . . I bottled that up inside me for a long time'. This is a feeling shared by many parents and does not mean you are unnatural or cruel. It is a good thing to talk about such feelings.

Talking about feelings does not mean you have to act on them.

Sometimes, parents repress this thought because they fear that to talk about it might lead them to hurt their child, or lead other people to believe that they will. In fact, talking about it makes it even less likely to happen, especially if your listener understands why you have such thoughts and can help you to understand too.

Blame and Anger

You always wonder why, why has it happened to us? Why wasn't it someone else?

Father of hydrocephalic boy

When you are faced with something you would rather not know, one of the easiest things in the world to do is to *blame* someone else for it. You might say your child is disabled because 'they' did not take proper care when she was born. Another parent might blame the school or the therapist. We do this kind of thing because we don't like our own feelings. If parents feel anger towards their handicapped child (but know she can't help the way she is), they often turn their anger towards someone else. Perhaps they pick faults in another child or have rows at work.

You can cope with anger by saying – I feel angry and bitter. These are my feelings. It hurts me that my child is disabled and there is no cure. And the hurt makes me angry.

Blaming others will not help. Your relatives and friends, and others who could help you, are powerless if you insist on casting blame.

Sadness and Despair

The need to feel angry, or to reject the results of doctors' or psychologists' tests will pass. Angry, rejecting feelings are usually followed by *sadness, even despair*. This is when you really face up to the fact of your child's permanent disability. You may feel worse than you have done since you first heard the news. You may wonder if things will ever come right. In fact, they are beginning to. In a way your sadness is the first sign that you are really accepting your child.

People learn to cope with sadness. We all have had our disappointments, our tragedies, but we learn to live with them and find that life has its good sides too. The danger is that the natural feeling of sadness can get mixed with depression caused by feelings of *shame and guilt*. Shame because you expect other people to think badly of you or your family. Guilt because you somehow blame yourself for what has happened.

Although attitudes are changing fast, some people will never understand that having a child with special needs has absolutely nothing to do with 'bad blood' in the family. We can choose our friends though, and ignore the ignorant. Having a handicapped child is nothing to be ashamed of and most people know that.

Feelings of guilt are more difficult to deal with. You may understand that your child's problems are not your fault. But because she is your child, you may feel that her problems are your problems, or that her problems might be less if you were better at helping her.

It is really unpleasant to feel this way. What parents sometimes do to try and stop themselves feeling guilty is to make a great show of doing everything for their child. They buy the child expensive toys and clothes, they devote great chunks of their time to caring for the child, feeding her and dressing her long after she could be doing these things for herself.

It is very tempting, though, to do too much for your disabled child. Sometimes parents *despairingly* feel that they cannot accept their child. They may wish she had never been born. We are taught that it is unnatural not to love our children, so we start to think that if we hate them, we must be wicked. We don't want people to know that. We don't even want to know it ourselves. So we forget it and we *make* ourselves love the child. In fact, we may smother the child with hugs and kisses, keep her away from all possible harm, feed her only mushy food in case she chokes, and so on. We make the child dependent on us, and we become dependent on the child to stay as she is so that we can go on caring for her. Because if we stop, we will have to deal with those feelings of rejection and dislike.

Some of the parents who act this way don't understand that it is natural to go through a stage like this. But, do remember,

You don't have to feel loving towards your child all the time. You don't have to be good and competent and happy all the time.

A mother of a physically handicapped boy had come to understand this feeling of 'being human' when one day she burst out, 'If he drops his spoon once more I think I'll explode!' At the time, she was talking with a social worker who was able to help her accept that it was all right to feel frustrated. Later in the same interview, the mother summed up her feelings when she said, 'It really helps to get these things off my chest. I know I won't really lose my cool if he does it again. It helps a lot to know I don't have to be Mrs Perfect Mother all day long'.

Again, it helps to talk about what you are feeling with someone who can help you understand what it is all about. Parents sometimes fear that if they think about or talk about their bad feelings at all it will lead to bottled up feelings bursting out. Then, they fear all sorts of problems, from marriage break-ups to being unable to carry on at all. In this case, you should remind yourself that you always have control over talking about your own feelings. You can let them out a little then choose to stop and then, when you're ready, let out a little more.

During this despair stage, it may be easier for a mother to talk about her feelings and to cry, than for *the father*. He may spend as much time as possible at work, or away from home, not realising the real reason for doing so. He may have had to support his wife and may now be feeling in need of some support himself. If this father is you, don't feel it is a sign of weakness to ask for support now. Many fathers of handicapped children are doing so and getting great benefits from it. As a mother of a multi-handicapped pre-schooler put it to us, 'I've let it all hang out with you, but my husband hasn't. But now after four years it's really got to him and he's really low. I wish he could have told me that before because I've been feeling OK about her for a while now and I think I could have helped him cope.'

Emptiness

Despair is sometimes followed by a *strange, flat, empty feeling*. You may look at your child and say, 'Well, she's handicapped. She can't do this and she won't do that, but there's not much we can do about it. We must just do the best we can'.

Realism and Hope

This is where therapists or teachers who can show you how to work with your child can make a big difference. We hope this book can make a difference too. They can all show you what can, with patience, be done. What can, with training, be achieved. Slowly, you begin to realise that your cup is half full, not half empty. You begin to feel more competent. You recognize even a tiny improvement as the success it undoubtedly is.

You realise that life goes on – and has much to offer, outside your home and away from the immediate needs of your child. A balance returns to your life and you find you are coping with demands at home, and can enjoy other activities too. You may always carry the sadness that your child is disabled, but you try to make the most of life for her – and for yourself.

Her brothers and sisters have come through it. You have been able to tell their teacher how to handle the situation if another child taunts them about their sister. You have learned how to stand up to the doubts and denials of any of your relatives or friends who find accepting her more difficult than you do. You have looked, in an adult way, at the problems and how they affect your marriage and your family, and you are finding solutions.

Elizabeth Straton
David Straton

BONDS

How do parents really become parents? It's fairly obvious where the process begins, but no-one hands out certificates that say you finally made it. Because *bonding* – 'getting in close touch and keeping in touch' with our children – never really stops.

However, creating this tie isn't all up to you; nor is it all up to your child. Parenting involves a partnership, and it takes two (parent *and* child) to get it together. In this part of the chapter, we will discuss what is involved in the important process of bonding and how you could help it to occur between you and your child.

Building a Bond

Recently, we've heard more and more about what needs to happen (or not happen) for the bond between a mother and her child to be firmly established when the baby is born. Valuable suggestions about how conditions should be changed in our hospitals so that this bond is not disrupted are backed by a certain amount of scientific evidence. This evidence points to the presence of certain hormones in both mother and child that appear at 'critical' times and help get the bond between them off to a strong start. It also indicates there are certain things parents and their new babies do most readily at these times if given the chance – things like looking at and touching each other – that help strengthen the bond.

Sometimes it may sound as if something automatically clicks into place and, from then on, the tie created between parent and infant is a once-and-for-all guarantee that they'll keep on giving each other lots of satisfaction.

This is not true, for even it the 'right conditions' (and we're still finding out what these are) are present at the beginning, this does not guarantee that the bonding is complete. Does this sound depressing? It's really just the opposite because it also means that even with the 'wrong conditions' to start with chances *are* still there for a parent and child to get started in developing their own special relationship.

It is possible for you to go on developing a bond, or close relationship, with your child indefinitely. And you can do this as slowly or as fast as is right for your child's and your own skills. **In other words, we don't accept the idea that if bonding doesn't happen at an early stage you've somehow 'missed the bus' and there are no second chances of it happening for you and your child.** There's no denying that it needs greater efforts on your part if it's been hard getting started, but as we find out more about what bonding involves, more can be said to parents about what they can do to help it along.

What do we mean by bonding? It includes what parents and their children *do*. People can make it happen; it's not just a mystical something that happens to them if all goes well. The idea we want to get across is this: babies begin very early to look, move, smile, cry, and make other sounds. Once your baby's behaviour and yours mesh or dovetail together, you have developed a bond or tie. This link-up comes about as each of you 'fits' what you do into what the other does. Sometimes the fit is better than at others, but it tends to improve as you get to know each other better. If your child's senses and skills are still developing, you are there to 'translate' her world to her – putting her in touch with you and, through you, with all that's going on around you both.

Bonding isn't Easy for Everyone

So far, we've stressed the positive and hopeful things about getting to be a parent. But there are many ways in which bonding does get disrupted or is made harder for some families.

Quite a few parents – mothers as well as fathers – don't feel especially close to their baby when she is born, and sometimes for quite a while afterwards. This isn't what we're usually told about becoming a parent – especially the first time around – but it can happen for a whole lot of reasons.

Some of these reasons are involved with what is happening when the baby's born – in labour, at delivery, and just after birth. Others have to do with how a parent is feeling. Also, the state the baby is in – her health, or how alert she is, or how much she cries or sleeps – can make it much harder to feel close to her.

But all three – the setting, the parent (s), and the baby – really go together in a sort of circular chain reaction, which can make becoming your child's parent an easier or harder task.

For instance, you may already know that certain anaesthetic drugs given to a mother in labour will suppress her baby's suckling for about four days. Baby and mother will both be drowsy and slow, so every kind of contact between them is damped down. And yet *physical contact* – touching and holding – as well as *eye contact* are really important at this stage to help trigger off the body reactions and the feeling in parents that draw them closer to their child.

So far we've talked generally about all kinds of babies and their parents. Every baby is born with needs to be satisfied, but each year some are born with special needs. If one of these children is yours, getting in touch can seem almost impossible. You may feel confused because you don't feel attracted to your baby. Or this confusion may be crowded out by stronger reactions more difficult to cope with – such as the ones we discussed in the first part of this chapter.

Building up a Relationship with Your Child

Bonding is not, as we said before, all up to you. You should be aware that the ways parents respond to their baby *are* affected by how she responds to them – the sort of 'cues' she gives them that show what she wants to happen next.

A baby who seems unresponsive is much harder to get in touch with. Where *are* these cues for you to pick up? Your own best efforts to make contact seem to get no results – 'She never seems to need me!' some parents tell us. Or you get results you neither want nor expect. You may even feel you have only a 'blurred' picture of your child as an unpredictable and confusing little being. What can you do?

☐ The first thing is not to expect too much too soon – of your baby or of yourself. Simply feeding, cuddling, stroking, looking at her, smiling and talking to her may or may not be hard for you to do, but they're the best start you could both have.

☐ In the very early stages of development – no matter what her age – it can be hard to pick up her responses to you. You learn to do this more easily in two ways:

(a) Watch what your child is doing . . .

To pick up the (sometimes very tiny) **signs from your child to which you can respond you need to become a very keen observer of her behaviour.**

This isn't as easy as it sounds. It takes practice, and it's helped greatly by some help, support, and feedback on how you're doing from a more experienced 'observer', as well as from your partner or someone else close to you. Some of the later chapters in this book can help too.

(b) Observe what *you* do, too. For instance, how quickly or slowly do you move, speak, start or stop actions? How smoothly or jerkily do you move her about, change her position? The pace and smoothness of your actions towards her can be a measure of your own tension level, which in turn can affect your baby's responsiveness – and the bond between you and her. If you are strung too high – or too low – it's probably harder for both of you to pick up each other's cues. By thinking about your own behaviour, you may decide there are changes *you* can make that could benefit you both. For example, do you give your child *time* to –

☐ take her turn with you when you talk or smile?
☐ get used to how something is feeling – by maintaining the contact long enough?
☐ notice how something is sounding – by letting the sound 'hang in the silence'?

By doing things with care and effort that seem to come naturally to some babies and parents, you begin to get to know each other better. You find yourselves a little closer, and perhaps a bit more relaxed more of the time. Moments of interest, fun – even excitement – begin to come more often. And the more in touch you are, the more general stimulation your child gets by touching, hearing, looking at you and the world you bring close to her.

This process is a bit like a spiral staircase. Each stair takes you a small step up *and* a little way around – two progressions for the effort of one. So it is with the stimulation you offer your child: it helps the bond between you grow stronger *at the same time as* it helps her own development. And of course, as her development moves on a step, she's just that much more capable of getting in touch with you and keeping in touch longer, which in turn makes it easier for you . . . .

To Sum Up:

☐ *Strong feelings are normal, don't be ashamed of them.*

☐ *You need to talk about how you are really feeling.*

☐ *Perfection is impossible — don't try to be superhuman!*

☐ *Bonding — building strong relationships — with your child is vital.*

☐ *Bonding is best started early, but it's never too late.*

☐ *Get in tune with your baby.*

Mary Lane

3 Growing and Developing

Many people think of a child with special needs in terms of his disabilities or his handicap – as someone who *can't* do things. It is better to think of him as someone who is *capable* of achievement and who *does* do things. Certainly, these achievements may take time and lots of repetition to accomplish, but they do occur. There are very, very few children who are incapable of developing any skills, however basic they may be.

How can you help your child develop his maximum potential? A good start is to understand some basic principles of teaching and learning. Five of these 'rules' are summarised in this chapter, and another two in the next chapter, making seven altogether. These rules are very important and they will come up again and again throughout this book.

Experiences need to be Planned

Children with special needs often have great difficulty in easily taking in the things happening around them – particularly if they have a major intellectual handicap. Because of this, there is little to be gained from simply bombarding them with stimulation. So our first rule is that these children *need carefully planned experiences*. It is important, therefore, that you decide on exactly *what* it is you want your child to learn and *how* you are going to teach him.

Development follows an Orderly Sequence

In deciding what your child could or should be learning,

remember the second rule: *development follows an orderly sequence, step by step.*

When he's ready to learn something new depends on what he can do now. For example, a child normally rolls, crawls, stands and walks – in that order. He learns to reach first by stretching his arm towards a toy, then by grasping it with all his fingers, and eventually by controlling the use of his hand well enough to take hold of the toy between thumb and forefinger.

This principle of development is very important when it comes to deciding what you should be helping your child to learn. It is much more important to ask 'What is my child ready to do next?' than to ask 'What should my child be doing at this age?'

Skills are Related

What should I be helping my child to learn? Although he will gradually be developing skills that seem quite different from each other – such as feeding, communicating, thinking, toileting, and dressing – it is important to remember that they are in fact related. For example, think about a child *listening* to a spoon rattle on a plate, actually *seeing* the spoon and plate, and then beginning to *link* these experiences in his mind. Or think of the connection between *seeing* how a toy works and *talking* about how it works. *You can't divorce these various skills from one another*, even if you have to teach some of them separately – our third rule.

Make the Steps Small

How should I teach? What's the best way I can help him learn? The fourth rule to remember is that *most skills to be learned should be broken down into a series of very small tasks.* For example, think back on how you learned to drive a car. First of all you probably learned how to steer it. Then you learned how to get into first and second gear – perhaps in a carpark on a quiet Sunday. And then you progressed to third and fourth gears on the open road. Now you can 'put it all together', almost without thinking. Remember this when you are teaching your child the skills of dressing, riding a tricycle, or feeding himself.

This rule of 'thinking small' is particularly important for children with special needs. Most children learn things so quickly that we don't even think of it as learning. It just seems to 'happen naturally'. Watching a child with special needs develop, however, is rather like seeing things happen in slow motion. He often has to be taught things bit by bit. You may have to break down a skill or task into several small steps and teach each step very carefully and in the right order. In the rest of this book, we will be suggesting ways of teaching like this.

If you set your sights on small steps you will find that your child is actually achieving things – a realisation that will bring you pleasure like that reported by the mother of Tony, a cerebral palsied youngster: 'Each little milestone feels such a tremendous achievement. I remember the first time he rolled over. I just picked up the phone and rang everyone.' Or the mother of a multiply-handicapped boy: 'Jess was just a little vegetable in the first 18 months of his life. He just lay there and looked – at nothing. I went through a tremendous period of depression. We hit rock bottom. It was only his first reaction that brought us out of it. When he reacted this was the biggest thrill we had in our life.'

Observe Your Child

To make the previous four rules work, we have to add a fifth one: *observe your child*.

☐ You must observe your child to understand his present level of development and to find the behaviour that tells you where he's at. For example, when he reaches for an object, does he *open his hand?*

☐ You must observe him to see if he can already do various actions that you hope to combine to make up a new skill. For example, if you wish to teach him to feed himself, see if he is able to hold a spoon and if he uses his fingers to carry food to his mouth. After all, he does need to know where his mouth is!

☐ You must observe him to see if he carries out the action you are trying to teach him. For example, how often does he successfully take his pants off by himself? Be sensitive to even the slightest progress.

☐ And as you will see in the next chapter, you must observe him to see if your idea of a reward (eg. a smile, a raisin, a cuddle) really is rewarding to him. Does he show any signs (however small) of pleasure or satisfaction when you give him any of these?

By observation, then, we mean *gathering a factual record of your child's behaviour.* It's much more useful to be able to say, 'He managed to get a spoonful of food from the plate to his mouth five times in five minutes' than to say, 'He's not very good at feeding himself'. After all, tomorrow he may manage ten spoonfuls in five minutes!

All this observation might sound a bit too much like putting your child under a microscope. (It may also sound like a lot of hard work – the kind scientists or teachers have to do, not parents). But, once you start trying it, it's actually a great way to get to know your child better. You start seeing him doing things you'd no idea he could do – and that can be very exciting!

So Remember:

☐ *Your child's experiences need to be planned by you.*
☐ *His development will follow an orderly sequence.*
☐ *His development will occur in various skills which are related to each other.*
☐ *Make the teaching steps small.*
☐ *Observe, and write down what your child does.*

David Mitchell

4 Encouraging Progress and Discouraging Mistakes

What Would You Do?

Let's start by asking you how you would deal with certain things your child might do. For each question there are five answers to choose from in the box below. Which answer (or answers) do you think would be the best?

1. Your three-year-old child cries hard every night unless you stay with her. Even after you've had a story together she still wants you to stay and talk. You'd like her to settle down after a story, without this long performance every night.
    Would you do A, B, C, D, or E?
2. It doesn't often happen, but your noisy two-year-old for once plays quietly while you're on the phone. This is something you want to encourage.
    Would you do A, B, C, D, or E?
3. You're trying to get the dishes done in time to keep a doctor's appointment. Your one-year-old baby is on her tummy on the floor nearby. Suddenly you see her fingers close round a spoon you've dropped and pull it towards her. (Up till now she's only been able to reach out and touch things, but couldn't seem to get hold of them or pick them up.)
    You're pleased; she's done something you want to see more of. But you're also pressed for time.
    Would you do A, B, C, D, or E?
4. Your eight-year-old child is always coming into the living room interrupting and doing things that get adults

to notice her when you're talking to your friends. Yet there are other children at home, and she and they usually like playing together.
Would you do A, B, C, D, or E?

A   Give her something she likes — a cuddle, a kiss, praise, a drink or a biscuit, more time to play or to watch TV, etc.

B   Leave her alone and pay her no attention.

C   Growl at her, or smack her.

D   Talk to her, and explain why she shouldn't do what she's doing.

E   Stop her at the outset with a firm 'No!', and immediately tell or show her clearly what you want her to do.

Answer: 1, *E* followed by *B*; 2, *A*; 3, *A*; 4, *E* followed by *B*.
At least some of these situations are familiar to almost every parent. They bring up some of the issues we'll deal with in this chapter, in which we will talk about two main rules – those to do with Reward and Punishment. In particular, we'll look at:

☐ encouraging behaviour you want
☐ using rewards to help your child learn
☐ how rewards work for parents, too
☐ discouraging behaviour you don't want.

ENCOURAGING BEHAVIOUR YOU WANT

Not Everyone Agrees about Rewards

Not all parents feel the same about responding to their children's behaviour. For instance, we asked one father if he thought praise was important for his child:

I think so. I like to be praised for something I do. I think it tends to make her try and do it right if you praise her . . .

But we also asked a mother what she does when her child does something the way she wants her to:

Nothing very much. I don't like this idea of reward particularly. It's fine with a dog or a cat or a horse . . . I'd rather keep prodding her along than have her do something purely for reward at the end . . .

By and large, we go along with the first parent. We do all tend to keep on doing things when the result is something that gives us pleasure — especially, perhaps, when the 'reward' was unexpected. If your wife tells you she likes the shirt you're wearing, you're more likely to wear it again. If your husband thanks you warmly for mending that leaky tap, you're more likely to do other things that please him.

Anything – however small – that gives us satisfaction, interest, comfort, or relief, will be rewarding. Ever since your child was born, you've been rewarding her in all kinds of ways, and – although you may not have thought of it this way before – your 'rewards' have helped her learn much of what she can do now.

Children Persist with Behaviour that has Rewarding Consequences

Remember the old game of 'Consequences'? At the end you had to say 'what happened afterwards . . .' Stop for a moment and think about the consequences of some of your child's behaviour. What happens *just after* she . . .

☐ throws a tantrum?
☐ has a good try at saying a new word?
☐ turns the handle of a closed door?

The consequence may be your reaction to her, or something she's made happen (like the door opening when she turns the handle properly). The point we are trying to make is that:

To help your child learn new skills, you can use rewards to reinforce her behaviour. Like steel rods in concrete, reinforcement is what makes something stronger. If you are 'strengthening' or reinforcing what your child does, it simply means she'll do it more often — and do it a bit better

each time. In other words, she'll be learning.

What is a reinforcer?
Anything that's rewarding for her can become a reinforcer –
a raisin, a bit of fruit, a lolly, a sip or a lick of something
sweet, a toy to hold or look at. It can also be something she
likes to happen – getting a cuddle, a big smile from you, or
being told you're pleased with her all help her to learn. It's
especially important that you *praise her even for the
slightest progress she makes*. After all, praise is communication as well as reward – and the clearer your message
the more easily she'll learn what pleases you.

Tell Your Child what Pleased You

What do we mean by praise?
What you say when you praise your child's efforts can teach
her a great deal.
So . . .
describe what she's done that you're pleased with. This is
the best way to get across to her exactly what you want to
encourage.

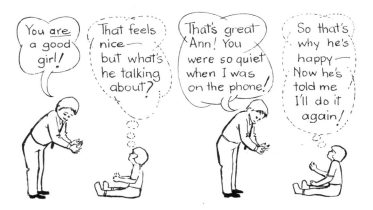

Figure 1   Tell your child what pleased you.

The Same Reward may not Satisfy Every Child and may not Satisfy the Same Child Every Time

What does your child find reinforcing?

Different children find different things rewarding. We adults may think something should be enjoyable for our child, but she may not think so.

For example, you may be trying to teach her to pick her clothes up off the floor, and decide to 'reward' her for this by letting her have a ride on a tricycle. But if she's really not interested in riding it, your reward will make absolutely no difference to her picking up her clothes. (And, if she's scared of being on the trike, it could even put her right off what you're trying to teach her.)

Here are three kinds of rewards that can be used as reinforcers. Choose some things your own child finds rewarding from each one:

☐ some small thing she likes to eat
☐ something she likes *you* to do
☐ something she likes to do *herself*

Obviously, any of these will cease to be rewarding if you use it again and again. So it's well worth trying out different kinds of reinforcers – things your child can find, or eat, or play with, or have fun doing. But remember, whatever other rewards you use, your pleasure at her successes is *always* important, both for her self-esteem and her continuing progress.

Reward Your Child's Successes

This brings us to our main rule in this chapter:

When she does something you like and want to see more of . . . reward her STRAIGHT AWAY.

Rewards Work for You, too

All these rewarding experiences sound like a lot of fun for your child (and so they should be). But what about you? Does it all sound like hard work on your side? You also have needs – for having fun, to be loved, to have your own efforts appreciated, and to have some time to yourself. Are your needs being met? If not, what can you do about it?

No-one can stay at the bottom end of the see-saw without everyone on it losing their balance. You must make sure you have ways of being rewarded too – otherwise you'll have nothing left over for anyone else. Plan your own rewards – big or small. Or, better still, work them out with your wife, husband, a friend (or two, or three), and your other children if they're old enough to co-operate. Look at what you might all 'give and take' (a word of appreciation, a favourite dessert, a hug, a half-hour without family interruptions, having someone else do a hated chore . . . . each of you knows best what makes you feel good). This way everyone looks after each other a little bit – and finds it rewarding too.

Helping your child learn will take time and patience. You and she may get confused, angry, frustrated. But give yourself time to appreciate what you have already achieved together. Then you'll also find that some of your own rewards are coming from getting to know your child better, and seeing her make progress because of your efforts.

DISCOURAGING BEHAVIOUR YOU DON'T WANT

What Would You Do?

1. Your child isn't keen on vegetables, but nor does she refuse to eat them. She's just learned to spoon food from her plate and put it in her mouth. One day you discover her carefully spooning vegetables from her plate – and on to the floor.
    What would be your first reaction: A, B, C, or D?
2. Your child is able to stay dry most of the time, but often wets her pants near you when you're talking with other adults.
    What would be your first reaction: A, B, C, or D?

3. Your child has burned her hands several times by touching the stove. You've erected a strong wire guard around it, but one day you come in and find she has pushed a chair close to this fender, and is just climbing on to it.
   What would be your first reaction: A, B, C, or D?

4. Over the last few days you've got your baby copying sounds you say to her. Today, she imitates you once, then grabs your hair or blows bubbles at you each time you try to get her 'talking' again.
   What would be your first reaction: A, B, C, or D?

A. Take no notice, so that what she's done won't be 'rewarded' with attention from you.

B. Tell her 'No!' firmly, and immediately show and tell her the right thing to do:

C. Explain carefully why she shouldn't do what she's doing.

D. Shout 'No!' and physically restrain her, (i.e. stop what she's doing by holding her or moving her away promptly).

(* remembering to praise her when she *does* start doing the right thing.)

Answers:
1,*B*;2,*A*(although, of course, you don't *continue* to ignore it – puddles need cleaning up and pants changing. But it's your *immediate* reaction we're talking about – see page 102 in the section on Dressing); 3,*D*;4,*A*.

There are times when you don't want to encourage certain ways of behaving. If you and your one-year-old want to play, for instance, you'll laugh, or pretend to cry, or blow bubbles back at her when she grabs your hair or blows bubbles at you. But this isn't what you want her doing at those times when you're encouraging her to make sounds that lead on to talking later. On the other hand, it's not behaviour that needs to be punished.

Some Things Should Just Be Ignored

Some behaviour that simply needs discouraging (like her 'inviting' you to play at the wrong time) can be reduced or stopped altogether if you and other people are able to take no notice if it occurs. Taking no notice can be hard to do, especially if you're feeling tense yourself. Sometimes (if you're up close and face to face) it's as simple as turning your head away, or making your face go blank and shutting your eyes. Sometimes it's just not saying anything.

'But it's not working!'

Some problem behaviour – like whining, tantrums, or head-banging – that your child may have shown for some time, may not stop when you try ignoring it. In fact, it may seem to get worse. For example, she may scream louder, more often, go on longer, or do it on occasions she's never done it before. IF YOU HAVE DECIDED TO IGNORE, IT'S ESSENTIAL TO KEEP ON IGNORING. Because if you pay attention to it after it gets 'worse', you've taught her that she can get your attention as long as she goes on long enough, or loud enough, or often enough. However, *this phase really indicates that ignoring is beginning to work, and that if you continue ignoring it and attend instead to behaviour you like to see, the unwanted behaviour can be reduced.*

Some Things You Can't Ignore

When your child is doing something like throwing a tantrum that's really hard to ignore, you could try this 'Time-Out' procedure: Say 'No!' firmly, calmly pick her up, take her to her room and tell her that when she's been quiet for a while she can come out. Only let her out when she's been quiet for the time you've said. (*Time her, and don't forget she's in there!*) When you go to get her, don't mention the behaviour that led to Time-Out, but help her to get a fresh start at some activity that'll quickly involve your encouragement and earn your praise.

Some Things Must Not Be Ignored

Don't be afraid to say 'No!' At times many children do need direct guidance from you to set them on the right course. What they're doing wrong rarely needs a smack or a scolding. But it does need stopping, with a clear 'No!' from you.

'*When I talk about discipline*', says one father of an intellectually handicapped four-year-old, '*I'm not talking about shouting and all that . . . As soon as she does something wrong, then I tell her to put it right, or I show her.*'

Punishment Does Have a Place . . .

Many people are confused about the question of punishment. There are certain times when it should be used – but by 'punishment' we do mean more than just smacking or growling.

What is punishment?
Anything that's NOT rewarding for her can become a punishing experience. *Punishment is whatever makes any behaviour stop* (or happen less often).

. . . But It's Not Much Use by Itself

Punishment may teach your child *to stop doing* something but it does not teach her what *to* do instead.

Punishment by itself is a short-term solution. But the effects don't last long, and after a while she'll be at it again. (Extremely harsh punishment can have lasting effects, of course – but the main one is that the child learns to avoid the person punishing her.)

Teach your child to avoid danger — teach her to avoid doing things that she really must not do but DON'T TEACH HER TO AVOID YOU.
The important point we want to make is that, after you've punished your child, for example, for running on to the road, be sure to make it rewarding for her to stay in safer places. You can do this by providing something more exciting for her to do, and THEN rewarding and praising

her for doing these things that keep her out of trouble. (Have you lots of ideas for play activities? If not, do you know where to find out more? The Supervisors at your local pre-school centre could help, and they welcome visitors to see what the children are doing. You'll find suggestions, too, in our list of 'Useful Books' in chapter 11.)

We All Tend to Stop Doing Anything that's Not Rewarding

There are two kinds of punishment. The first includes those where you make something nasty happen to your child – a smack, a growl, a fright. These are hardly rewarding experiences – *unless this is the only kind of attention she gets from you, in which case she may well find it rewarding*! The second kind of punishment is where you make sure that nothing nice happens for a short time immediately after she misbehaves. If nice things are already going on for her when the behaviour occurs, make sure you stop these rewards immediately. (For instance, if she's watching a favourite TV show, and starts hitting her little sister, don't hesitate to turn off the TV straight away and remove the other child quickly and quietly.)

Most times this second kind of punishment works well. The *absence* of a reward the child was expecting – losing some little privilege, or missing out on everyone's attention (and company) while she's in Time-Out – can effectively cut out a lot of inappropriate behaviour.

Being really firm doesn't have to include being angry or harsh (or feeling guilty afterwards!).

Punishment is a more complex matter than reward, so our final rule is not one simple guideline like all the others. Instead it's a package of seven essential points:

The Seven Rules of Punishment

Where punishment is needed, remember these pointers if you want it to be effective:
1. Do it IMMEDIATELY.
    Timing is just as important in punishment as in reinforcement.

2. Punish (wherever you can) by taking away rewards.
   These include attention from other people.

3. Make it clear how the child can get rewards again.
   *(When – and only when – she stops the unwanted
   behaviour).*

4. Punish CONSISTENTLY.
   *A behaviour may persist even if you punish it eight times
   out of ten but let her get away with it once or twice.*

5. Reinforce other behaviour you're happier with, to put in
   the place of the punished behaviour.
   *Otherwise the effects of your punishment won't last
   long!*

6. Use words to help your simple message get across.
   *'No, hot!' 'You don't go on the road!' – these tell her
   more than 'You naughty girl!'*

7. Stay cool – or as cool as you can.
   *Your child learns a lot by copying you. If you lose your
   temper when she loses hers, what is she learning from
   you – to do what she sees you doing, or to obey what
   you're telling her? (You can let off steam later, if you
   feel you need to.)*

Finally . . .

These rules can work for all children

You've probably realised by now that all we've said in this
chapter isn't just about children with special needs. These
rules are the keys to strengthening (or weakening) all kinds
of behaviour performed by all kinds of people – children
and adults.

Think about the others in your family. How could you
begin using these suggestions to make your home a more
rewarding place for everyone – including you?

Mary Lane

5 Feeding is More than Eating and Drinking

Your child will find learning to talk much easier if he can already breathe and eat properly. How is this? When you stop to think about it, speech, like eating, requires precise movements of the tongue, teeth, lips and other parts of the mouth. Therefore, eating is not only important in its own right, but will help your child to develop speech.

In this chapter we will be giving you some ideas on:

☐ the importance of feeding patterns
☐ finding suitable feeding positions
☐ preventing excessive dribbling and helping sucking
☐ introducing solids
☐ developing tongue control, jaw movements, and chewing
☐ encouraging drinking from a cup and through a straw
☐ preventing your child from manipulating feeding.

Feeding Patterns are Important

Almost all babies are born with an ability to feed. You can probably remember that right from the time your baby was born, if you touched his cheek, he instinctively turned his head in that direction and started to suck.

During the first year or so, most babies gradually learn to control their actions well enough to become skilled in eating and drinking. When they start taking solids at about four to six months, for example, it doesn't take long for them to learn to keep their lips closed round the food, and to use their tongues to push it about inside their mouths.

But you may find that your baby has more difficulty controlling the movements of his tongue, lips and jaw. He may take longer than other children to pass the usual 'messy' stage of learning to eat properly. This stage is not all that pleasant to cope with at mealtimes and you might be tempted to feed your baby before the rest of the family. But it is important for him to take his place at the table, with its conversations and opportunities to learn how people behave and get on with each other, and the sooner he can join you the better. Even more importantly, a lack of control of tongue, lips and jaw can eventually interfere with his *speech development*.

For these reasons, we think it is important to find ways of helping your child to develop good feeding patterns.

Find a Suitable Feeding Position

We suggest you do not feed your child when he is lying down, mainly because it seriously limits his ability to experience what's going on around him. Instead, sit your child in an upright position leaning slightly forward. Make sure he is comfortable.

Here are some ideas for finding a suitable position for your baby:

☐ Your baby can be fed facing you on your lap (Figure 2). Put an arm or a small pillow on the table edge behind his shoulders and neck. Try to keep his head upright. It is almost impossible for him to swallow if his head is tipping backwards or if it is sitting on his chest.

☐ If he is very floppy, he may need to be propped up with extra pillows. You could also try placing him in a child's car seat or a specially-moulded chair to fit his body. (Figure 3).

☐ You may prefer to sit your child sideways on your lap with his bottom between your legs. In this position you should support him by putting one arm around him at shoulder level, leaving one hand free to hold the food or spoon. (Figure 4).

☐ If your child is older, you may find he is more stable with

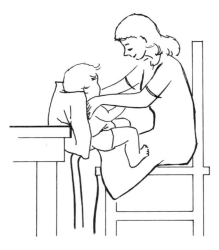

Figure 2 This is a comfortable position for your small baby.

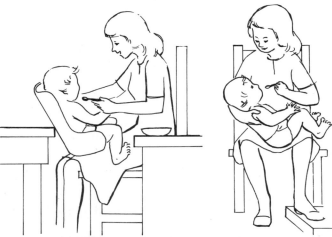

Figure 3 You could try other means of supporting your baby.

Figure 4 The position must be comfortable for you, also.

a table in front of him at chest height. This will enable
him to rest his arms on the table.

Make sure you are well prepared before you start feeding
your child. Have the food, spoon, a face flannel, and
anything else you will need ready.

In these early stages, when you are concentrating on
feeding your child or teaching him how to feed himself, try
to avoid distractions and make sure your other children are
occupied. When he has learned some good feeding skills,
you can be more relaxed and have him with you at the family
table. Whatever you do, remember to make mealtimes
enjoyable for both you and your child.

Prevent Excessive Dribbling and Help Sucking

Your child's lip movements are important, both for eating
and for speaking. If he can't keep his lips together, he will
dribble. If he has trouble in controlling his lip movements,
he may have problems in tightening his lips for sucking. If
this persists, he may have problems in making vowel sounds
such as [oo] or [o] and lip consonants such as [p], [b], and
[m].

Some children with special needs have difficulty in co-
ordinating their swallowing muscles, or in controlling their
jaws, or in closing their lips. This is particularly true of intellectually handicapped and cerebral palsied children, many
of whom dribble excessively.

There are various ways in which you can help your child
stop dribbling. Some of these suggestions apply to babies,
while others are best used with older children. Remember to
make these activities enjoyable for you both by talking and
joking as you do them.

☐ Try lightly moving your finger downwards on your
child's throat. (Figure 5a).

☐ You could also use circular movements on his throat.
This helps to stimulate the muscles used for swallowing.
(Figure 5b).

☐ Another way to help your child learn to close his lips is to
put your first finger between his top lip and his nose.
(Figure 6).

Now stroke down on his top lip two or three times. Next, put your first finger under his bottom lip and stroke upwards. Finally, gently pull on his bottom lip and let it spring back.

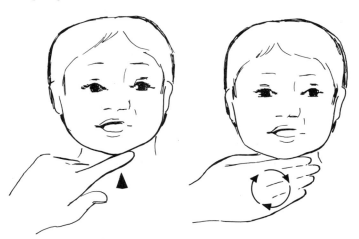

Figure 5a/5b   Stimulating swallowing.

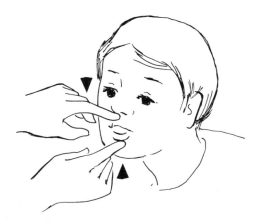

Figure 6   Both of these movements help lip closure.

☐ Blowing whistles or hooters or humming on a comb wrapped in tissue paper can help an older child to keep his lips together.

☐ If your child dribbles as a result of forgetting to close his mouth, a gentle tap under his chin or a touch of his lip will remind him.

☐ If your child is older, but still needs a bib, use a cowboy scarf or cravat. To make them, stitch an absorbent material between two pieces of material.

☐ Your child may not know when his face is wet. Help him to learn the difference between wet and dry by blowing warm air on to him from a hair dryer and talking about the different feelings of wet and dry. These concepts can be taught during bath-time or when you are washing the dishes or playing in water with your child.

☐ Teach him to use a handkerchief if he can manage one. Remember, your aim is for him to be as independent as possible.

☐ Finally, as with most of our activities, remember to

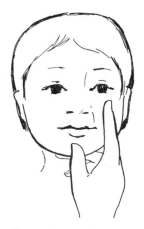

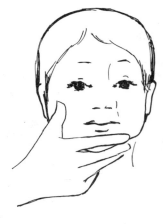

Figure 7a This position gives good support to his head.

Figure 7b Put your arm around your child's neck for support, and your fingers in this position.

reward him when he tries to swallow, and when his face is dry.

Note: If your child's dribbling poses a severe problem, surgery can help correct it. However, this is normally not considered before the age of five as there may be some improvement up to that age.

Help your Child to Chew and Swallow

Some children need help in learning to chew and swallow their food. Ways which we have found to work are shown here. In the first drawing, you will notice that you should place your thumb on your child's chin to keep it still. Your first finger is on his cheek and your middle finger is under his chin. An alternative way of arranging your fingers is shown in the second drawing. In either way you help your child to chew and swallow by:

☐ moving your fingers *on his cheek* in circles to help him chew.

☐ moving your finger *under his chin* in a downward direction to help him swallow.

Introduce Solids Early and Carefully

Most children begin to eat solids at around four to six months. For a variety of reasons, however, some children stay on a liquid or pureed diet for a longer period. Our view is that all children should move on to a solid diet as soon as possible. As we have pointed out earlier, this gives them more opportunities to learn to chew and eventually helps their speech.

What can you do to help your child eat solids?

☐ It could be that his mouth is over-sensitive. If so, he may gag or vomit on solid foods. This could be because he has never put his fingers or other objects into his mouth like most young babies. You could help this by giving him soft rubber animal toys, especially those with protruding parts such as bills, legs and tails. In general, too, you should not stop him from putting his fingers in his mouth.

☐ Your baby's mouth may be very tender. Stroking his gums might help here. Try to make a game of it as not every youngster likes to have someone's fingers in his mouth! With an older child you could pretend to be counting his teeth or looking for a loose one.

☐ As your baby becomes able to tolerate solids, introduce a variety of foods homogenised to the consistency of baby food. Gradually introduce foods thickened by potatoes, oatmeal, wheatgerm, etc, and then move to such foods as cottage cheese and mashed bananas. Eventually, he will be able to deal with foods of a mixed consistency, eg., stews and vegetable soup.

☐ When beginning to spoonfeed your child, only half fill the spoon and place the food on the tip of the spoon. Give small mouthfuls. If he doesn't open his mouth, open it half way and place the spoon on the front of his tongue. Press down firmly with the spoon and gradually withdraw it, allowing his lips to take the food from the spoon. Remember to close his lips to encourage him to move the food around his mouth, rather than pushing it out.

☐ If he clamps down on the spoon, don't force his jaws open but wait for him to relax before taking the spoon out. We suggest you use a metal or wooden spoon, but not plastic ones because they tend to break easily.

Do you know what to do if your child is choking on his food? It is unwise to hit your child on his back if he starts to choke because this causes him to inhale and can worsen the problem. Instead, move him forward into a bent position, supporting him by your arms. Put your fists under his ribs and give a quick upward movement. This will usually dislodge the food. If you react quickly and *calmly*, there will be no danger and your child will not be frightened. But do *take care*.

Develop Tongue, Jaw and Chewing Movements

Most children don't start chewing until around four to six
months of age. Children with special needs may not be
ready to chew until somewhat later. Some may open their
mouths too widely; some may have difficulty in biting their
food; others may be able to bite it but lack the control of
their jaws and tongue to chew it. It takes all children time
before they can bite and chew properly.

☐ To help your child learn to *bite*, place food such as a
strip of carrot between his front teeth and when he
begins to hold it pull gently on it.

☐ As you know, *chewing* involves using the side and back
teeth to grind food moved there by the tongue. You
could help him learn to do this by occasionally placing
food between the chewing surfaces of his teeth.

☐ Stimulate chewing movements by moving your finger
tips in circles on the outside of his cheeks (Figure 8).

☐ With an older child you can show him how to chew by
letting him observe you chew your food.

☐ Choose foods that are suitable for chewing. Dried fruits,

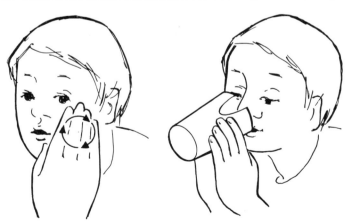

Figure 8 This circular movement on your child's cheek
helps chewing.

Figure 9 Try using a cut out
cup.

orange in a muslin bag, and thin strips of juicy meat are excellent foods on which to practice chewing. Food like white bread and buns often end up as a sticky dough in the roof of the mouth and can often cause a child to gag.

☐ Sometimes you might find that your child thrusts his tongue out of his mouth instead of chewing his food. If you are feeding him with a spoon you could help to control his tongue by pressing down and slightly back on it with the spoon. But do make sure you do this gently or he will gag.

Encourage Drinking from a Cup or a Straw

How can you help your child *drink from a cup?* Here are some suggestions:

☐ Begin by using a slightly thickened liquid which flows more slowly. This can be made by adding a little baby rice to the milk. As your child becomes more skilled, you could gradually thin the liquid.

☐ Try using a soft plastic cup with a rim that can be squeezed to form a spout. Place this spout on your child's lower lip, giving him small amounts of liquid at a time.

☐ Cut out a semi-circle about 2-3 cm (1 inch) down from one side of a plastic cup and let your child drink from the high side, leaving the cut-out piece for his nose. By using this cut-out cup, his head doesn't have to be tipped right back and swallowing is therefore easier. (Figure 9).

Drinking through a straw is a skill which normally doesn't develop until a child is three or four years of age. It helps develop the lip control so necessary for speech. Some ideas:

☐ A thick-walled plastic tube about 12 cm (5 inches) long makes an ideal straw. It lets only a little air up with the liquid, causing less painful wind. (You can obtain this tubing from Chemists).

☐ Place the straw on the middle of his bottom lip, just in front of his teeth.

☐ If he has difficulty beginning to suck, use a soft plastic bottle with a hole cut in the lid for the straw. Squeeze the bottle, allowing some liquid up the straw. Gradually reduce the flow as your child learns to suck through the straw.

Prevent your Child from Manipulating Feeding

Some children throw tantrums, refuse to eat, and generally manipulate mealtimes to get their own way. You will probably agree that this should be avoided, but sometimes parents react in such a way as to increase it. For example, if you scold or cajole your child to eat, you could well be drawing too much attention to his 'bad' behaviour. As we've mentioned in chapter 4, this attention often makes things worse.

These pointers might help you to deal with this problem, especially with an older child:

☐ Allow your child to decide himself whether or not to eat. Having made this decision, he has to live with the consequences. Almost all children will decide to eat when they are hungry. You cannot force your child to eat, but you can stop fighting with him about food.

☐ Serve small amounts with no comment about eating or not eating. Don't scold or coax him to eat. After 20 minutes or so clear away the food.

☐ If your child begins to eat his food, *praise him*. Gradually increase the amount of food you expect him to eat before you praise him. Eventually, only praise him when he has a clean plate.

A Final Word:

All through this chapter we have emphasized that by helping your child to develop good feeding patterns you will:
☐ *help him to eat appropriate food*
☐ *help him to develop the control of muscles required for speech*
☐ *help him to be socially acceptable.*
Feeding is much more than simply learning to eat and drink.

Christine Hilton

6 Communication is a Two Way Street

We have to use simpler words, but that's not very different for any child. Any child at that age you tend to use words that they will understand and have heard before.

Father of Down's Syndrome boy

I used to talk to her a lot. One thing we noticed because of her loss of sight was that she never smiled and this was a disappointment. But I just treated her like any other baby, as if she could see and hear.

Mother of deaf-blind girl

As adults we take language and communication very much for granted, but we are all aware it is an important part of our everyday life. We use language in different ways for so many purposes – to communicate our needs, to have discussions, to give commands, to express our ideas, to gain a greater understanding and so on.

Learning language is a very complicated business and no-one has all the answers as to how children develop these important skills. We can describe *what* children are doing at various stages as they learn language but we know comparatively little about *how* they actually learn it.

The first word is thought of by many parents as the beginning of language, but it is really just the tip of the iceberg. Before this great event a lot happens that actually paves the way for your child to begin using words. She must, for example, be able to hear, to listen, to distinguish between sounds, to associate particular sounds with certain things, and to build up an understanding of the language she hears about her. An understanding of language usually precedes your child's ability to talk and it is likely that she will always understand much more than she can express.

In the previous chapter, feeding patterns and their importance for speech have been emphasized. Here we will suggest ways you can assist your child's progress in developing language. We will look at:

☐ important points to bear in mind as you read through this chapter
☐ the early stages children go through in learning to communicate and use language, with ideas at each stage for ways you can help your child with special needs.

We have chosen to discuss language development in a series of stages because this is a convenient way of grouping together several things that are happening round about the same time. They are not rigid categories, and it is quite normal to find your child at one stage of development but still doing some things from the previous stage as well. Each stage builds upon things that have happened in earlier stages.

IMPORTANT POINTS

Language Development follows an Orderly Sequence

The development of language follows a pattern. Children progress through certain stages as they develop. Most research shows that children with special needs go through the same stages as other children. For example, they learn to pay attention to people, to imitate sounds, and to understand language heard about them, before they begin using words meaningfully. Although children with special needs go through the same sequence of development, they may do so at a slower, and sometimes at a much slower, rate. Specific handicaps can affect this development. Some children, for example, may never complete all the stages in language development. Many Down's Syndrome and other children will have difficulty with making sounds clearly. Sometimes, cerebral palsied children also find it very hard to express themselves; and while some of these children will have no problem, others will experience difficulties understanding what is said to them as well. A child with a hearing loss will not hear speech as others do and will be at a distinct disadvantage, not only in developing speech, but in developing an understanding through language.

Don't Leave It to Chance

It was once thought that by giving handicapped children a good stimulating environment they would eventually speak. We now know that this alone is not enough. Handicapped children – particularly those with language delays – need extra help. They need to be taught the skills of speech and language.

Make the Steps Small

Earlier, we discussed how skills may have to be broken down into small steps and each step taught in turn. This applies to teaching language, too. If your child is continually failing at a task, your steps may be too big for her.

Reward Successes

As we've mentioned before, make sure you reward your child straight away when she does what you want, no matter how small that achievement is. As her efforts to communicate improve, she'll often get a 'built in' reward. For example, when your baby makes gurgling, cooing sounds and you talk back to her and smile, she is being rewarded immediately for making those sounds by the interest you show. Later, when she says 'Drink,' and you get her one, she is learning that she can use words to get what she wants.

Look for Language Opportunities

Remember that in a book such as this one, we are able to

offer you only a few ideas. Look for ways of extending these ideas to suit your own child. Make the most of what is happening about you during the day and when you play together. You'll find a list of other books which offer language suggestions in chapter 11.

STAGES IN EARLY LANGUAGE DEVELOPMENT

We shall consider early speech and language development by looking at what happens as your child passes through various stages. What you have to remember as you read through these is that:

☐ Several things will be happening at once in each stage.
☐ Language skills are not isolated, but are closely related to other skills.
☐ The order in which your child learns things *within the stages* will not necessarily be the same order as we have listed in this book.

Let's begin at the beginning.

Stage I: Early Communication

From the time your baby is born, she has to cope with a wide range of different experiences and to make some sense out of them. She learns during this stage not only how to make some of her needs known, but also to respond to other people.

Cries have a Message

The first sound your baby makes as she enters this world is the birth cry. The air floods into the lungs, filling them. The air is then pushed out again, the vocal chords tighten up, and the first sound, a cry, is made.

At first it is doubtful if your baby knows exactly why

she's crying, but as the weeks go by you will notice changes in her cries. They become more precise signals of her needs.

What are the Different Ways your Baby Cries?

☐ There is a cry of pain which you can hear from the first day onwards.

☐ There is a cry which tells you that your baby is hungry, uncomfortable or cross.

☐ Later there is a 'happy cry' which is often referred to as 'cooing'. Sometimes it sounds like cooing but at others like grunting, gurgling or squealing.

You may find it difficult to tell the difference between cries and to know exactly what your baby wants. Some of the time you'll feel you're learning very much by trial and error. Nevertheless, when your baby cries and you respond, together you are building the beginnings of communication. Remember – communication is a two-way street.

Babies Pick up 'Conversational' Clues

Conversation-like sessions between parents and their babies actually begin before the 'cooing' cry develops. Your baby picks up clues which affects the way she reacts to you. These are picked up from:

☐ your voice – it can sound comforting, angry or happy, and so on

☐ your facial expressions – the way you smile or frown at her

☐ how you handle and touch her

It is easy to think of your young baby as being helpless, and in many ways she is, but there is much she can do from the first few weeks of life. For example, films of adults and babies show that babies are often 'in rhythm' with adults speaking to them. They make movements of their bodies, their arms and their heads. A baby and mother will keep looking at each other as the mother speaks. At first, the baby may not make any sound during these 'conversations'. Later she begins experimenting with lip and mouth movements which are similar to the movements we make when we speak. Communication is being built up as the sounds and gestures which your baby makes get reactions from others.

Babies Learn to take Turns in Conversations

Before long, one of the most interesting things that happens is that babies learn that you have to take turns when having a 'conversation' with someone. They will respond to their parent's talking and smiling by smiling back. With your own baby it is important to give her that chance to 'have her say'. When she responds to you, keep looking at her but wait until she almost finishes smiling and moving before you begin talking and smiling again.

If your child is severely handicapped, you may have to really 'work' at getting a response. Keep talking, smiling, singing and playing. It's easy to give up, to forget, because you don't get a response. Keep trying and look for little signs like eye movements, a concentrating expression, a stillness, which alert you to your baby's efforts at getting in touch with you. Encourage every effort she makes.

These communication skills are happening in part because your baby is learning to understand the sounds and sights around her.

Help Your Baby to Learn through Listening

From birth, your baby hears sounds. Sudden noises will usually upset her, making her jump, shudder or cry. She will show that there are some sounds, particularly soft ones, that she finds pleasant and others that she dislikes.

You may notice that your voice is one of the most effective ways of soothing your baby when she is upset. Before long you will find her turning to your voice more often than to other people's voices. She is associating your voice with things she enjoys – being picked up, changed, fed, bathed . . . . With this awareness, she will begin listening more and more to the sounds about her and experimenting with sounds she can make herself.

Let's look at ways we can encourage listening:

☐ Make different sounds with a bell, a rattle, the radio, a whistle, a drum and see which ones your baby likes.
☐ Sing to her.
☐ Put her outside where she can hear different sounds.
☐ Vary your voice as you speak to your child – whisper, make it louder, softer, higher, lower.
☐ Introduce noise-making objects into her mobiles – foil milk bottle tops, little bells, keys that jingle.
☐ When your child is sitting on someone's lap or propped up, try ringing a bell gently, out of sight behind her head. Does she turn to look for it? Play this game at different times, using a range of toys which make different sounds. Vary the position where you make the sound – first on one side, then on the other. Each time your child turns to the sound show her the object and praise her for finding it. (See Figure 10).

Is Your Baby Hearing?

Deaf or partially hearing babies may not be disturbed by sudden loud noises or show the same interest in sounds as other babies. It is, however, just as important for them to see your mouth moving as you speak.

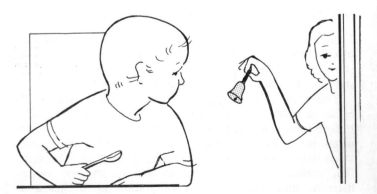

Figure 10   Encourage her to listen.

If you are at all concerned about your baby's hearing, or if she is not making sounds when you feel she should be, ask your doctor for a hearing test. Some children have what is called a "fluctuating" hearing loss. At times they can hear well, but at others they miss out on a lot that is happening around them. This is particularly true of Down's Syndrome children who are likely to have colds or respiratory conditions which may affect their hearing. If your child is deaf, seek help early. Your doctor can refer you to a specialist or speech therapist or you can go through one of the larger organisations for the deaf.

Help Your Baby to Learn through Looking

Your baby's eyes are one of her first means of finding out about people and objects in her world. During this early communication stage, she learns to recognise familiar faces and movements. She begins paying attention to people and things rather than just 'seeing' them. She learns to connect what she sees with what she hears. At first she will only be able to focus on objects that are close – 20 to 60 cm (8 to 24 inches) from her eyes. She can 'see' objects further away than this, but this ability is generally limited to seeing contrasts between light and dark or between sudden changes in light. As she develops she will be able to focus on objects more accurately and for longer. She begins to inspect things with her eyes – especially your face and her hands. She begins to search for sounds with her eyes, indicating an increased awareness of language and what is happening about her.

Here are some suggestions for developing your baby's looking skills:

☐ Provide plenty of opportunities for your child to see faces. Initially put your face close to hers so that she is only 20 to 30 cm (8 to 12 inches) away. Encourage other members of your family to do the same.

☐ It is most important that your baby learns to focus her attention on your mouth and what it does. Later this should help her to learn the way sounds are made during speech. Sing and talk to your baby, at times exaggerating your mouth movements.

☐ It is essential for later learning that your child should pay attention not only to people, but also to objects. Hang simple mobiles close to her bassinet, her changing table or where she lies on the floor. Make them by using everyday things you find around your home – colourful cards, yoghurt pots, small toys, a woolly ball, a small circle of carpet. Your child will look longer at things that have pattern, texture or depth than at simple, plain flat things. Because of her interest in human faces, draw a rough picture of a face, or cut out a magazine picture, and use it on your mobile. (See Figure 11).

☐ When you are carrying your baby, don't always go whizzing past things. Occasionally stop for a few minutes and give her a chance to look. Talk to her about what she is looking at.

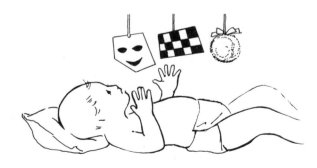

Figure 11   Develop your child's looking skills.

Stage II: Experimenting with Babbling

Why is 'Babbling' Important?

Babbling is an experimental stage in language development. It's the time when your baby really starts experimenting with all the 'apparatus' she has for producing speech – her mouth, tongue, vocal chords, lips and the various muscles involved with them. Most importantly, she learns how to gain control and to co-ordinate this apparatus so that she can produce a wide range of sounds. Let her have quiet times on her own when she can carry out this playing with sound.

At first, the babbling sounds she produces are the ones she finds easiest to make. They are vowels and consonants which become connected in long strings of sounds, for example [ba-ba-ba], [ma-ma-ma], [da-da-da]. Listen to your baby; she is not simply imitating sounds she hears you making. Indeed, you would find it difficult to imitate her, for many of the sounds she is playing around with are not used in our English language at all. As you give her more attention when she makes sounds which are close to the words we use, she will discard some of the earlier sounds, but by then they have played a vital part in her speech development.

Children with a hearing loss begin babbling in the same way as other children. But as time goes on, the sounds they make do not become more like the speech sounds used about them. Instead, by about 11 or 12 months of age, the quantity and range of sounds they produce will become noticeably less – unless they are given special help.

Increase Babbling

Although your baby will only rarely imitate the sounds you want her to make, you can encourage her to increase the *amount* she babbles. As your baby's ability to make sounds grows, she will become more aware of other sounds. She will often stop when she hears a voice and listen before she begins babbling again.

The following ideas can also be used with older handicapped children. (With the older child it is important to encourage all speech-like sounds so that you have a base to work from in developing speech).

□ Speak gently to your child, and keep looking and responding when she 'talks' to you.

□ Touch her chin gently. This has been found to increase babbling in some babies.

□ Sit with her in front of a mirror so that she can see her mouth moving while she makes sounds. Make sure she can see your mouth moving too as you talk to her.

□ Tape some of your baby's 'talking' and play it back to her at different times during the day.

□ Use language in a variety of ways. Play 'Peep-Bo' and other games which are played around the fingers and toes like 'This little Piggy Went to Market'. These games help your child associate language with a pleasurable activity and at the same time assist her develop an awareness of her own body. With an older child look for fingerplays and games which are more suited to her interests.

Stage III: Understanding, Attention and Imitation

During this stage your baby:

□ Gains more and more *control over people* around her by drawing attention to herself through sounds and actions.

□ *Learns* a great deal, not only about the world around her, but also about language as you *play* and *talk* with her.

□ *Copies actions* and *sounds* and *understands* more and more of the language she hears.

Your Baby Learns to 'Make Things Happen'

Up until now your child has had little idea of what makes things happen. Gradually, often by accident, she comes to find out that she can act with a purpose (or intention) and make things occur herself. For example, if she hits a squeaky toy it will make a noise. If she cries, babbles loudly, or calls out, people will take notice of her. She realises that she has some control over people around her through her sounds and actions. It is important that you encourage her growing understanding by responding to her. Mind you, she may make her demands so clearly heard that you would have difficulty ignoring her anyway!

Understanding Language Comes Before Speaking

Your baby has already learnt that sounds are different. Now she is learning that different sounds stand for different things. Remember how earlier we said that your baby learns to understand language before she uses it. At this point, important skills of language understanding are developing:
☐ She begins to understand that sounds refer to objects, people or actions.
☐ She begins associating particular words with a particular object, person or action.
☐ She shows in a number of ways that she understands the meaning of some of the language she hears about her. For example, she will look towards the door when you say, 'Daddy's coming'. She will stop doing something when you say, 'No'. She will point to a named object when you ask her to.

Encourage Understanding

Your child must be able to understand language before she speaks with understanding. Try these ways of encouraging understanding:

☐ Talk about your child's toys as you play with her. Roll her a ball and say 'ball'. Use the word in short sentences. Sometimes hold the thing you are naming close to your face so she looks at your mouth as you say the word. She will see the ball, she will hear what you say, and eventually she will link the word and object together. Play lots of naming games with her.

☐ Look at picture books like the *Ladybird* series. These have good clear pictures of things found about your house. So. .e intellectually handicapped children have difficulty at first in understanding pictures. Show your child the real thing – for example, a spoon – then show her a small spoon (perhaps out of a doll's tea-set), and later show her the spoon and a picture of it together. Make it fun.

☐ Encourage your child to look at objects when you point to them. At first she will watch your hand. Move your finger slowly until it touches what you're pointing at. Teach her to point. You may have to help her point with her first finger many times before she gets the idea.

Can she follow simple commands? See how many she can understand:- 'Wave bye-bye', 'Give it to me'.

With an older child, you can encourage many movements:- 'Sit', 'Stand', 'Shut the door'.

With these activities, you are encouraging your child not only to understand language but also to pay attention and to begin imitating you.

Encourage Attention and Imitation

Imitation plays a crucial part in learning to speak. A child must be able to imitate actions, sounds, and later words. She must be able to remember many things before she can imitate. Imitation, or copying, is not a skill that comes automatically to children. It is one that is learnt. With many children it has to be taught and it can take time. Before your child can imitate she must be able to pay *attention* to people. How can you encourage this?

☐ Sit down in front of her with your head at her level and say 'Look at me'. Does she look at you? If she does, reward her with a small amount of food or drink that she likes, or a smile, a hug or a clap. Repeat this over several days until you can guarantee that she will always look directly at you when you give this command. To make it more interesting, sometimes show her a special favourite toy when she looks at you. If your child does not look at you, place her face between your hands and direct her gaze at you while saying 'Look at me'. As soon as her eyes are looking at yours, show her in some way how pleased you are. Gradually give less and less help. If you are rewarding her with food or drink always smile and praise her as well so that this becomes the most important thing to her.

☐ Once she looks at you when you request it, teach her to respond to her name when you are further away from her. Call her name. Does she look at you? Does she keep looking at you as you speak to her? If the answer is 'No', get someone to help you teach her. While your baby is not looking at you, stand at her side slightly behind her, and call her name. If she doesn't respond when her name is called, get your 'helper' to take your child's chin and gently turn her head to look at you. Gradually give less and less help. Once your child starts turning to her name on her own, smile and praise her.

☐ Try calling her from several different positions in the room. Always remain visible. Show her you think she's great when she finds you. Encourage other members of your family to join in this game, too.

Once your child looks at you when you call her name you can teach her to *imitate actions, movements of your face and, later, sounds.*

☐ Teach her actions such as clapping her hands, raising her hands above her head, waving goodbye, banging a drum . . . Here is an example of how you could teach her to copy an action:

(i) Prop your child up with cushions or sit her in a chair. Sit in front of her. Clap your hands. If she does not copy you, take her hands gently and clap them for her. Talk to her about what you're doing, 'Clap, clap, clap your hands'. Make it fun.

(ii) Stop. Clap your hands again. Help her again, holding her hands very lightly. If she makes any attempts at movements with her hands, smile at her.

(iii) Continue in this way, gradually giving her less help at bringing her hands together. Continue to smile and to praise her every time her efforts to clap improve.

(iv)   When she gets the idea and starts clapping, lighten your touch until your child is clapping her hands by herself. Show her how pleased you are.

☐ Move now to the face. Encourage her to copy you when you move your face – opening her mouth, putting out her tongue, licking her lips . . . . These actions may prove more difficult for your child as they are not actions that she can see herself performing. Make use of a mirror. *Remember, you don't always have to be the leader*. Copy what she does, too.

☐ Once she can copy actions, the next step is to see if you can get her to imitate sounds. Listen carefully to the sounds she makes. Pick out a sound that is close to the one we hear in everyday language. When she makes the sound, copy her. Make sure she can see your mouth. At first, reward *any* attempts to make a sound. If your child makes no response, shape her lips with your fingers as you make the sound. Try a wide variety of speech-like sounds. At first your baby will find the vowel sounds [a], [ee], [oo], [i], [u] and the consonants, [p], [b] and [m] the easiest to make.

☐ With your older child, play with toy animals. Make the appropriate noise for each animal, encouraging your child to join in. Animal noises contain many of the sounds your child needs for later speech. Gradually, she will imitate more of the sounds you make and her babbling will sound more like adult speech.

Play is Important

We can see now that so many of the skills we have already discussed – listening, looking and imitating – are all coming together. Added to these is the wide range of play experiences your baby is having. Through play she will be learning and developing ideas about things around her. For example, she begins to associate the word 'Teddy' with the play-thing that she has pushed, pulled, thrown, chewed and cuddled.

As she develops ideas about objects around her, she has less difficulty in associating words with them.

> Children with severe physical handicaps often have less chance to explore through play. They need more assistance from you. If your baby is physically handicapped, you may need to take objects to her, help her to find out more about them, how to use them appropriately . . . Allow her the chance to see, hear, taste, smell, touch and move a wide variety of toys and things in her environment.

Stage IV: First Words

During this stage, your child's understanding of language develops at a rapid rate. She begins imitating some of the words you've used frequently with her. She learns to use between 10-20 words correctly. In the beginning, these words are used for naming things. Then she realises that they can be used to make things happen or to stop something happening. If she calls 'Mummy', mummy will come to her. When she says 'No!' strongly enough, people understand that she doesn't want to do or to have something. When she begins using words in this way, she has reached a new stage in her development. She is beginning to take part in real conversations with you. There are many things that you and all your family can do at this point to increase your child's understanding and help her develop language skills. Think of ways of extending the ideas below:

☐ Teach your baby to point to familiar objects in a book as you name them. See if she can find the page with an object you name on it.

☐ In the bath, name her body parts as you wash her. Encourage her to point to the main parts.

☐ When you are dressing her, talk about the different items of clothing.

☐ Play games with her toys. Ask her to give them to you as

you name them. Ask her to get something familiar from another room.

Stage V: Putting Words Together

A most dramatic step occurs in your child's communication when she begins putting two words together. At first, these two-word 'sentences' are probably imitations of something you've said, ('Good girl', 'Bye Daddy'). But then you will begin to notice her saying things she obviously hasn't heard before, ('All-gone ball', 'All-gone book', 'All-gone Teddy'). In these examples, she is attaching a variety of words ('ball', 'book', 'teddy') to a certain 'pivot' word ('all-gone'). This use of a pivot word marks an important development because she is now showing that she understands how words are related to each other. This awareness will be great fun for your child and you will probably hear her practising her two-word sentences over and over again. Give her time to practise on her own without interruption.

But it can't stop with two words. One of the problems of two-word sentences is that they often have several meanings. For example, 'Daddy car' might mean any one of 'Daddy's in the car', or 'That's Daddy's car', or 'Where's Daddy's car?' or 'Let's go out in the car' – depending on the circumstances. It's only when she starts putting three or four words together in sentences that her meaning can become clear. Even then, she will still leave out some words, but those essential for getting her meaning across will normally be present, ('Daddy go car', 'Me go home').

You can encourage your child's use of two-word sentences, (and eventually three-, four- or more word sentences) in a variety of ways:

What Words is Your Child Using?

Keep a list of the words your child says. Are they all naming words or are there some *action* words (verbs) like 'jump', 'go', 'sit', 'eat', 'book'? Does she use any *social* words like 'bye-bye', 'ta', 'no', 'yes'? Does she use any words that tell you *where,* like 'up', 'here', 'there', 'down'?

If you find your child is using only naming words, you need to look at ways of encouraging her to use more words from other groups, otherwise she won't have enough of the words she needs to put together into sentences.

Increase Action Words

Action words, or verbs, are essential if your child is to develop more mature forms of language:

☐ These are best taught by showing the child the action, (or by naming an action she already does), and then having her make the movements herself. Talk about what you and she are doing. At first you may get only a one word response, 'eating'. Increase this to two words, for example, 'Mummy eating'.

☐ Play action games with dolls. Give commands – 'Make dolly sleep'.

☐ Find pictures in magazines of people sleeping, washing, walking, drinking. Make them into a scrapbook that you can talk about, using two word sentences – 'Baby sleeping', 'Boy washing' . . . .

☐ Take photographs of your child doing various things. Include these in the scrapbook.

Increase Words that tell 'Where'

Use similar ways for teaching 'where'. Remember that at first a child must use real objects and be able to put objects in different places (in, under, there) during play before he can understand these ideas in pictures. You can also make use of pointing when teaching 'here' and 'there'.

Use a Range of Techniques

☐ Increase the number of words in your child's sentences by slightly expanding what she says. For example, when she says 'Man jumping', you could say, 'Yes, the man is jumping'.

☐ Use questions as a means of encouraging more language. Just watch that you don't continually ask questions. They should be used occasionally. Your child will understand 'what' questions first, and later those beginning with 'where', 'how' and 'why'. Once you ask a question, always respond to the answer she gives.

☐ Expand your child's use of language by using words she has already to express new ideas. For example, she may say 'Daddy run' and you can expand this to 'Yes, he is getting the ball'.

☐ Continue enjoying books together. Use those with a lot of repetition such as 'The Little Red Hen', 'The Gingerbread Boy', 'The Elephant and the Bad Baby'. Encourage your child to 'join in' wherever she can on the familiar repetitive phrases – 'leave room' for her to take a turn rather than rushing on with the story yourself.

Communication can Occur Without Speech

Some children with special needs will always experience great difficulty in communicating by spoken language. Over the last few years, some such children have been taught successfully to use sign systems devised for deaf people. In many systems the signs are used along with the spoken word so that the child continues to see and/or hear the words at the same time as they are seeing the signs. Although these systems have limitations, they can reduce many of the frustrations associated with language difficulties.

Other means of communicating by body language, gestures, written words and pictures may also need to be taught and used more extensively with certain children. If you are at all worried about your child's progress in talking, seek help from the people we have suggested in this book.

Remember:

☐ *Communication always needs at least two people.*

☐ *Communication is more than just speaking.*
☐ *Understanding generally comes before speaking.*
☐ *Looking, listening and play are essential for language development.*
☐ *Attending and imitating are essential steps on the way to understanding and speaking.*
☐ *Keep talking to your child, even if progress is slow.*

Jill Mitchell

7 Learning to Think

When he's lying in his pram we always move him to where the action is.

Father of spina bifida boy

Obviously this is what you've got to do isn't it? If you're not getting through in one way you change don't you?

Father of Down's Syndrome girl

When we are thinking, we might be remembering, planning, putting things in order in our minds, working out problems or making decisions. These are all 'thinking skills' which we use to cope with life's demands. We began to develop them very early in life – from infancy onwards, in fact.

In the past, few people expected handicapped children to be able to learn like other children, and they weren't helped to develop these skills. But much research, and patient effort by parents and teachers over the years, has made us realise that almost every child *can* learn, given the right experiences. Now we try to give them all thinking skills which will:

☐ help them learn ways of coping with the demands of their world
☐ give them a sense of their own worth through success
☐ help them achieve their full intellectual potential.

We also know that the way parents handle and stimulate their baby or young child can make a big difference to how easily he learns to think.

Progress depends on *your child* and his ability to learn, *his environment*, which provides opportunities for learning, and *your ability to help* him make the most of his opportunities.

Your Child Learns to Think through Play

Your child must learn to look, listen, handle objects properly, move about purposefully from place to place, communicate, and understand his world if he is to cope with it. He learns to do this by gaining control of his body, practising his skills, understanding how to make things work for him, exploring new materials, and trying out different ways of using things. Adults call this play. In fact, it is the child's work; his business is *to learn – through play*.

There are Stages in Learning to Think

Like all children, he will move through a series of developmental stages or steps, changing from a helpless baby to a youngster who is on the road to independence. For some children that road may be very short, for some very long, but all need to be helped to start their journey upon it. And that's where you come in. He needs you for comfort and closeness, reassurance when things go wrong, praise when he succeeds or improves – however slightly.

So you need to know what is an improvement. That means you need to know what he can and cannot do. As we have explained in chapter 3, good observation is the key here. Do you know which developmental stage your child has reached in his thinking and how to help him reach the next one? We hope this chapter will help you to answer 'yes' to both questions.

STAGES IN LEARNING TO THINK

In the rest of this chapter, we will go through the early steps of development in detail and make suggestions for creating a good learning environment for your child. As you can see in the following diagram, we will be discussing six stages – starting from birth and going up to what four year-old children achieve.

Ages have been included in this chapter to give you an *approximate* idea of when *most* children learn to do certain things. If your child is handicapped, it is likely he will take considerably longer to learn some or all of these skills; *it is very important that you do not try to force your child to learn things before he is ready*.

CLIMBING
UP THROUGH THE
EARLY STEPS OR STAGES OF DEVELOPMENT

6	*Taking apart and putting together, Putting things in order.*	6
	It fits here! Matching colours, sizes, shapes.	
5	What happens when I do this?	5
	Understanding my world; words go with things.	
4	*Developing attention – control.*	4
	I like doing this – I'll do it again. Hide and seek	
3	games. Things in books. I can copy you.	3
	Where did that noise come from? Reaching for and	
2	*grasping objects. Basic manipulative skills.*	2
	Early stimulation of movement and all the senses. Making	
1	a relationship – somebody loves me.	1

Figure 13   Stages of development.

The First Step (Developmental Level 0-4 months)

Learning how to cope with the world starts at birth with breathing, sucking, closing our eyes against bright lights, moving our limbs in unlimited space. At that time, your baby has to react to things that happen to him – but he can also make his own needs known. He makes his presence felt – and life for his family is never quite the same again! As parents, you will need to learn how to recognize and respond to his demands for food, warmth, and rest. You can also recognize when he is ready for learning and respond by giving him an appropriate environment and plenty of stimulation.

Stimulate Your Child to Look

In the previous chapter we have discussed ways in which you could help your child to develop 'looking skills'. You will recognise many of them as common games that adults play with babies. Often, however, parents do not play them if their baby is handicapped because they don't expect the baby to respond. Keep trying – he will. Here are some additional ideas you could try out:

☐ Bend close to him as you feed and change him (20 – 30 cm or 8 – 12 inches) and try carrying him in a front-pack. He may not be able to see much while he is very tiny, but the *contact* will be extremely valuable in creating a bond between you.

☐ Train him to *follow objects with his eyes* by painting a red and yellow bullseye or a black and white chequer pattern on a piece of flat wood or thick card. Hold it 20 – 30 cm (8 – 12 inches) from his face and jiggle it until he looks at it. You may need to jingle a bell with it to attract his attention. Then move it from side to side, up and down, and round in circles. Do this several times a day until he is good at it.

It is better if he is in a flexed position while you do this – lying on his back with his head supported by a cushion, and another cushion under his legs. Very young infants or physically handicapped children may be more comfortable lying on their sides, although this will clearly restrict the amount of eye-following they can do.

☐ Ask another person to help you teach him to *glance from one face to another*. Hold him up so that he can see your face. Have the other 'face' about 60 cm (24 inches) away on a level with yours. First get him to look at you and then ask the other person to attract his attention. Then call him back to look at you – and so on. You can do this with objects or your patterned cards as well. It helps him learn to control his eye movements.

☐ Move him from room to room and put his cot in different parts of his bedroom. *Make sure he always has something interesting to look at.* Remember – when he is very young, he will prefer strong contrast between light and dark. A little later, he will be keen to watch you and others as you move about the room.

Stimulate Your Child to Listen

Ideas for stimulating your child to listen may be found in the previous chapter, Communication is a Two-way Street.

Stimulate Your Child to Touch

In this first stage, he will be aware of *textures, temperatures* and *pressures* against his body. He will be able to move his hands to touch his clothes and face, and we can encourage his awareness in many ways:

☐ *Hold him* close and let him feel your face, and the rise and fall of your body as you breathe, cough or laugh. *Blow gently* on his face and other parts of his body.

☐ *Rub his body gently* with a towel, a clean nappy, a piece of silk or velvet, a crumple of soft cellophane or tissue paper.

☐ Let him feel different *textures* – cloth of various sorts, sheepskin, fur, hide, leather, polystyrene, wood, sandpaper, and so on.

☐ While washing him, use a firm rubbing action especially on his back from top to bottom. Let him feel the soap and bubbles. Drip some water on to different parts of his body. Splash him gently if he likes it.

☐ Think of ways to introduce him to differences in *temperature*, warm and cool. Put a warmed spoon on his cheek and some cool drops of water on his face and hands. Hold him close to your own warm body.

Remember to talk to him about what you are doing.

Stimulate Movement in Your Child

As you well know, your baby can move his limbs and trunk from birth. You might also have noticed that if he is startled, his limbs will fly apart and his back will arch. If he is cuddled, his body will relax and 'cuddle in'. If you put your finger into his hand, he will grasp it. These movements can be extended in a variety of ways:

☐ Pick up your child and *cuddle him* frequently. Try to make a point of doing so, not only when he is upset and you are hassled yourself, but also when you are feeling relaxed and happy. Encourage him to relax, and take up a cuddled-in position, with no stiffness in his limbs.

> **It is extremely important that you help your child learn good positions to be in. A physiotherapist will help you with this.**

☐ Carry him around, so that he learns what *movement* feels like.

☐ Get him used to lying on his *stomach* and to different positions.

☐ Move his bassinet around so that the light from the window or electric light falls on him from different angles. This encourages him to *change position*.

☐ Prepare for *head control* by strengthening his shoulder and neck muscles like this: lie him on his tummy on a large beach ball or bolster and roll him back and forth, holding him by the ankles and supporting him with your hand on his back.

☐ Encourage him to *lift up his head* when he is lying on his tummy, by putting your face at his level and calling him, or attracting his attention with toys. If his head seems too heavy, lift it for him by raising his chin gently and stroking the back of his neck and, as his eyes meet yours, smile and blink and tell him how pleased you are. When he is looking at you, see if he can hold his head up himself by removing your hand from his chin. Expect him to manage this only briefly at first, but praise him or do something he enjoys as soon as he is successful even for a second, and repeat this exercise several times a day.

□ Help him to *grasp* your finger or other small objects. If his fist is tightly clenched, gently tap the back of his hand with your outstretched finger in a downwards movement and, as his hand loosens, slip in your finger.

This first stage is his introduction to the sights, sounds and sensations of his world. It is a preparation for later stages. You have been preparing him to use his senses effectively, and to bring them under his own control. His response to stimulation is partly something all babies are born with – *a desire to be active* – but increasingly it will depend on how his environment responds to him. In the early days, you are a crucial part of his environment and, throughout his early childhood, it will be your reaction that counts, as far as he is concerned. So show him he is loved for himself, and that his achievements, however tiny, are appreciated. Encourage his efforts to communicate with you. Get to know how he expresses his needs and how you can satisfy them. (See what we've said about reinforcement in chapter 4.) Your reward will be an increasingly alert and responsive child who is on the way to thinking.

The Second Step (Developmental Level 4-8 months)

Your child is now going to broaden his horizon. His sight matures so that he can focus clearly on you across a room. He can distinguish between sounds, responding to such things as approaching footsteps, sounds of meal or bath preparations, and friendly or disapproving tones in your voice. He will learn to reach out and grasp an object and transfer it from hand to hand. He will be able to watch what he does with his hands, and he will learn basic manipulative skills such as waving, shaking, banging his toys and dropping one in order to take another.

During this stage, you can continue all of the activities of stage one that you both enjoy, but introduce some new ones:

□ Attract his attention from across the room. Encourage

him to *follow* your movements with his eyes. Smile and talk to him when he notices you and calls to you.

☐ When he is in a supported sitting position, hold up an attractive toy within his reach. Help him *reach* for it and take it by raising his arm at the elbow and putting his palm in contact with the toy. Praise him when he succeeds. As he becomes more able to reach, make him stretch and persevere to reach the toy, but never to the point of frustration.

☐ When he is holding a toy, encourage him to play with it by bringing his other hand to it, and *transferring it from hand to hand*.

☐ Show him how he can *bang, wave* and *shake* a toy.

☐ When he is holding a toy, offer him another and encourage him to *drop* the one he is holding in order to take it. If necessary, knock the first toy out of his hand with the second, as you slip it into his now empty hand.

Remember not to pull his arms and hands forward as this may make him want to resist you and pull back. If you feel any resistance in his arms, or if he pulls back, seat him so that his shoulders and back are supported and you can manipulate his arms from behind him, so that you are easing them forward by gently pressure from behind, not pulling from in front.

The Third Step (Developmental Level 8 – 12 months)

Some very important thinking skills begin to emerge now:

Children Learn to Make Things Happen

Firstly, your child will find out how to make an interesting event happen again. He might knock a cradle gym with his foot quite by accident rather than design, but the result will please him and he will try to do it again. This signals a big improvement in his ability to control his own body, his recognition of events going on in his environment and what he can do to make them happen. He also learns how to use his voice to attract attention. Make sure your child gets a chance to *make things happen* for himself during this stage. If he wants your attention, give it. You can then easily attract his attention back to toys (unless he is tired, ill or hungry), which will allow you to get back to your work. But if you ignore him, he will not learn that he can make things happen when he wants to, and will give up trying.

Children become Aware of Object Permanence

The *second* major thinking skill to develop during this step is his awareness of *object permanence*. What this actually means is that he realises objects still exist even when he cannot see them. This knowledge will let him learn to think about things not actually present, i.e., things in the past or the future. At a more practical level, it will allow him to remember where things are, and go and find them! As we've mentioned in the chapter on communication, object permanence also enables him to understand language, so that when he hears a word, e.g., 'cup', and sees an actual cup, he will learn to link the word with the object.

Children Learn to Imitate

The *third* skill is more of an aid to learning than an actual intellectual skill. It is *imitation*. Your child learns to imitate familiar actions and then quite new ones. At first, he might copy you picking up a block and waving it. That is a familiar action to him. Later, he might copy you picking up a block and dropping it into a box. Dropping is a new skill and he will have to work out how to copy your actions with his own body. Again, in chapter 6, we have pointed out how your child copies sounds you make, at first ones which are already in his repertoire and then new ones. How can you encourage these important thinking skills to develop?

☐ Provide him with *toys that move* when pushed or pulled, make a noise or change in some way when he touches them. A 'busy board' with knobs to pull, switches to push, dials to turn and little doors to open gives him plenty of interesting things to repeat.

☐ Help him learn to *pick up* tiny objects with his thumb and forefinger, and to use his index finger to explore things like dials, faces, switches and clothes fastenings.

☐ Encourage him to *copy you* tapping a spoon on a cup, blinking your eyes, making sounds and pouring water in the bath. Think up lots of new actions for him to copy and make a game of trying one new one every few days.

☐ Partially hide a small toy he is playing with under a cloth and help him *to find* it again. When he is competent at finding a partially hidden toy, hide it completely and let him pull away the cloth to find it. Move the toy to a different hiding place and help him find it again. Hide another toy under a box and then cover the box with a cloth and encourage him to keep looking. Such games develop object permanence skills and lead the way to your child being able to *remember*.

During this stage, your child has acquired the foundations of some of the most important skills involved in thinking and coping. He will now be prepared to begin understanding what you say, and learning ways of looking after himself.

The Fourth Step (Developmental Level 12 – 20 months)

Develop Understanding through Curiosity

During this period, your child's mobility and general awareness of the world will mature so that he can become much more *curious* about what happens around him. Instead of repeating what he has done before, he will begin to search for new ways of doing things with both new and familiar objects. For example, given an egg-beater for the first time, he will attempt to find out all its possibilities, turning the beaters with his fingers or turning the handle, whereas before he might just have banged it on the ground or used it in the same ways as other objects. Now, however, he looks at each thing as if trying to learn about its particular properties. It is as if he is learning to understand the nature of things in his environment and how each may be used.

Your Child Learns how to Attend to Tasks

At around this time, another change occurs which can make him appear more difficult to handle. It is partly that he wants to do things for himself. But more importantly, he is developing *control of his own attention to tasks*. He has to learn to ignore all the other things happening around him in order to concentrate on what *he* chooses to do. At first, it is very difficult for him to manage and he cannot tolerate your efforts at 'helping' him by talking or showing, 'look at me, look at how I do this . . .' He sees you as an interference which must be cut out. You may think him obstinate unless you understand his need to learn to direct his own attention. Sometimes he gets so frustrated by his inability to do what he wants, and by you trying to make him do what you want, that he may throw a temper tantrum, or slide onto the floor in a floppy heap!

Either way he has succeeded in cutting himself off from the task which is causing him frustration, but he's also preventing you from helping him learn. Unless you can find a way to change this sort of behaviour and persuade him to be more co-operative, he may not develop many new skills for several months.

Keep Your Child Making Progress

What can you do to change this? One way is to wait until he is older, but to give him toys appropriate to his developmental level to play with as he wishes. When he is older and can understand what you want him to do, he may be more likely to co-operate. If you do decide to wait, choose appropriate toys and activities from the suggestions which follow and show him what to do by playing alongside him. For example, if you want him to build with blocks, give him some and build with your own on the floor next to him where he can see you. Modelling rather than pushing often improves co-operation.

You can also try to provide learning tasks that you do not have to 'explain' to him. An example of such a task would be a little box with a loose fitting lid, into which you slip a raisin, then cover the raisin with a block and put the lid back. The child, who has seen you put the raisin in, is then prepared to take off the lid, remove the block and get the raisin. Also, try a formboard with easily removable circles with large-headed drawing pins stuck in, so that the child can slip them in and out of their holes easily.

> This technique may be sufficient for mildly handicapped children, but those who are finding it more difficult to learn to control their own attention and to develop new skills will probably need a more determined effort on your part to overcome their negativism and keep them progressing. This will take some skill – and lots of patience, so don't begin until you are well-prepared, and fairly sure of what to do.

Help Your Child to Co-operate

The first thing to do is to *choose an appropriate task* – one that your child is ready to learn. You establish this by reading through the activities suggested in the steps described in this chapter, and seeing which ones he can already do and which ones are still way beyond him. In between these and the ones he already manages will be the tasks that he is ready for.

For example, one grandmother who looked after a mentally handicapped three-year-old told us that once her grandson Michael could bang a spoon on his high chair, she taught him to tap a toy xylophone with it. Then she showed him how to tap the xylophone with a square block. From there she got him to tap the block on a second slightly larger block, and showed him how to let go of it there. After that they added another block on top. Soon Michael was building 'towers' of 3 or 4 blocks. Granny was successful because she started with a skill the child had already learned – banging the high chair, and used it to develop new skills –

first, tapping a xylophone – second, placing one block on top of another.

Although she didn't know it, Granny was successful because she also used other techniques which are valuable in helping children learn. Let's look at some of those techniques.

After you've chosen a suitable task, *the next step is to set up the situation so that your child will be able to attend to the task and learn.* This means that you must:

☐ Choose times when you and your child are relaxed and able to spend time on the task in hand when you aren't tired or hungry or in a hurry. You *are* looking forward to doing something together.

☐ Plan to spend between three and six sessions each day working on your chosen tasks. Make each session no longer than five or ten minutes.

☐ Make sure you have everything you will need within your reach (but not his!) before you start.

☐ Make sure you will not be distracted – take the 'phone off, put the dog out, remove other toys and children (if possible), switch off the radio.

Granny used the time after meals to teach Michael, as he was always co-operative then. She had time after morning tea, lunch, and afternoon tea. She removed the meal things, fetched the necessary toys and turned Michael's chair to face the wall, so that he could 'keep his mind on the job!'

When you've set the scene for learning, *you next need to let him know what you want him to do.* So first, be a model for him – show him the things you're going to use, and demonstrate what you want him to do. Keep it simple – if you want him to bang a tambourine then just pick up the tambourine, bang it and put it down. Nothing more. If the task is to put blocks into a box through a hole in the lid, then place the box where he can see it, and drop two or three blocks through, one at a time. That's all.

Now comes the difficult part – you must *secure your child's co-operation* in learning the task.

☐ Teach him to respond to certain requests and let him

know straight away that he's done the right thing. For
example – first get his attention:

'Michael, look' (He looks at you) 'Good look, Michael'.
'Michael, take' (He takes the block you are offering)
'Good take Michael'.
'Michael, put block in' (He puts the block into a
container) 'Good put, Michael'.

☐ Get him to respond correctly by *shaping* his actions,
using your hands to show him what to do – like this:

'Michael, look' (turn his face towards yours and praise
him as his eyes meet yours, even if it's only the merest
glance at first. You may have to practice getting his
attention in this way many times before going on to the
next request). Don't forget to praise him for each little
success.

'Michael, take' (put your hand on his hand to help him
carry out the action). Praise him.

'Michael, put block in' (use your hand on his hand to
help him carry out the action). Praise.

☐ As he learns what to do, gradually remove your hand
from his until your hand is just close enough to *prompt*
him if he falters.

☐ Finally, *remove your prompting hand altogether* so that
he responds to your spoken request alone.

Michael's Granny found that sometimes it worked better if
she sat *behind* him so that he couldn't pull his arms out of
her grasp, especially the first few times she tried anything
new.

Another good way of securing his co-operation if he tries
to 'act up' is to put both his hands flat onto the table,
cover them with your own, and turn your face away from
him for about a minute. Just hold his hands down still
and give him no attention until he settles down again.

One father told us how difficult it was to get his deaf-
blind daughter to co-operate. She would scream and wriggle
furiously until he felt like hitting her, and had to just walk

away and leave her. So he and his wife decided that she would hold the child from behind, sitting at a low table, and he would 'shape' her responses with his hands on hers. They did this many times a day, just for one or two minutes each time. They worked on teaching her to reach out and feel things, and praised her all the time.

After many *weeks* she began to sit quietly and allowed her father to move her hands. After several *months* she began to respond by reaching out as he requested – and so they learned that she was perhaps not totally deaf. Two years later she went to a school for blind children, where she is doing quite well.

Finally, a word about praising – or *reinforcing* – the behaviour you want. The technique is discussed more fully in Chapter 4, so the only things to add here are these:

☐ When you praise your child as part of teaching him to attend and learn as described above, ('Good look, Michael' . . . 'Good take, Michael') we suggest you use this form of words because it is very specific, and your child will come to understand what you mean.

☐ Strengthen your message by smiling and touching your child in a way you know he likes.

☐ Give him a tiny taste of something he likes at the same time, if you feel you aren't progressing well enough by using spoken praise and smiles alone.

☐ At the same time as you are removing your prompting hands and letting him do the action by himself, try leaving off the 'tiny taste' and some of the praise, so that you only reinforce him every so often. For example, if he's building with blocks, praise him after the third one and, say, the fifth one goes on, and when he's completely finished, rather than as each block goes on.

Michael's Granny found that he loved marshmallows, cut into four pieces – he had one piece each time she needed to use a 'tiny taste'. He also loved tangerine segments, and – of all things – cashew nuts. When he got older he liked being allowed to play with a car that shot rockets as a reward. What does your child appreciate most as a reward?

Developing attention control as a part of learning new skills can take several months, during which your child will require firm, consistent handling, especially since this is likely to be the period you are teaching self-help skills such as eating with a spoon. Mastery of such skills is very important to your child's sense of self-worth, so do persevere, with patience, through what can be an awkward time.

Here are some activities to encourage different thinking skills at this stage:

☐ 'How do I make it happen?' Try and give him something new to handle every day – different kinds of paper, tin foil, ribbons, a handbag, a balloon, a tin with stones in it.

☐ 'I can use this to make it happen'. For example, show him how to reach a toy by pulling a string fastened to it. If he won't grasp the string, fasten it to his wrist for a while and let him feel it jerk the toy as he moves his arm. You could also make a ramp by placing a piece of board against a chair. Show him how to slide toys down when he is sitting and pull them up again with the string.

☐ 'What does this thing do?' To help your youngster learn about the properties of things, you could:
— look for opportunities to let him play with different kinds of musical instruments,
— let him explore gadgets such as an old typewriter, an old telephone, old alarm clocks,
— give him chances to do 'messy' play with flour, sand, thick paint.

☐ 'I know where it's going'. Learning what happens to objects when they move is an important skill in young children. They can be helped to learn about this by:
— rolling a ball from one to another,
— putting objects in and out of containers,

☐ 'You make it go for me'. Sometimes your child might want to know about how things work and will hand it to you to make it go. Try to encourage this.

☐ 'I can copy you'. Copying what someone does is a good way of learning some things, so:
  — help him learn how to copy gestures like waving bye-bye or putting his hand on his head,
  — see if he will copy you when you ring a bell or put beads into a box.

Children Learn the Idea of Causality

During this stage, your child has been learning the basics of *causality* – if I do this, then that happens. This not only provides him with much information about how the things in his environment behave when he handles them, but also allows him to decide *what to do* and *how to do it* – essential skills in learning to cope with the world.

The Fifth Step (Developmental Level 20 – 30 months)

Children Learn to Solve Problems

In this stage, your child becomes capable of *planning with foresight*. That is, he begins using what he already knows to solve simple problems. Suppose he wants to open a door, but his hands are full. He can now work out a way of doing it: either he stands and shouts, knowing someone will come and open it for him, or he can put down some of his toys, open the door, pick them up and carry on through – problem solved! Simple, but important in coping with the world at his level.

Help Your Child to Remember

He also begins to remember things that have happened in such a way that he can *recall* them for use in an appropriate situation. This may not always be convenient for you. For example, suppose you are out in the supermarket, and he sees another child 'throwing a tantrum' to get a packet of raisins which his mother does not really want, but for peace she gives in. A couple of days later, at home in your kitchen, he wants a biscuit just before dinner. You refuse and wham

– there for the first time is a tantrum just like the one he saw! Hopefully, you will ignore it and he will learn that behaviour like that does not work with you.

Another time the telephone will ring when you are hanging out the washing. By the time you reach it he may already have answered it – and hung up again, saying 'Bye for now' just like he's heard you do so many times!

He can also use his new powers of recall in more useful ways. He might consent to put away his clothes or fetch things from another room, and he can begin to learn to dress himself because he can remember not only what part of his body his clothes fit but also the sequence of actions it takes to get them there.

Help Your Child to Experiment

In these and other ways, recalling useful ways of doing things in a new or different situation is a very valuable coping skill. It allows him to *experiment* with a fair idea of what might happen, which is a more mature way of solving problems than the trial and error methods he has used previously. His manipulative skills will now be good enough to allow him to use more difficult equipment and to experiment to see how it works.

He will try to think out solutions to the problems presented by the equipment. He needs plenty of practice and so we have grouped activities under five headings, each dealing with a different kind of thinking, or problem-solving:

☐ 'Playing hide-and-seek with toys'. In this activity, your child learns that a toy still exists, even when it is hidden. Get his attention, then:
— Hide a toy in a small box, then cover the box with a cloth. Let your child find the toy. Repeat this, but move the box to beneath a second cloth, leaving the toy under the first cloth.

☐ 'How do I solve this little problem?' Learning what effects he can have on things around him is an important realisation for your child. You can help this by playing games like the following:

— Give him a tall container like a plastic drink bottle with a long thin necklace inside. See if he can get it out and then work out how to get it back in.

— Give him some wooden or plastic rings to stack onto a piece of dowel. Slip one or two solid shapes of similar thickness and colour into the pile and see if he rejects them.

☐ 'What can I do with this?' To help your child become interested in what he can do with different playthings, give him plenty of chances to sort and arrange things. For example:

— Give him an opportunity to paint with a large brush. Use thick, bright paints and large sheets of paper (newspaper will do). Fasten the paper securely to the floor or on an easel,

— Give him a plastic tea set and encourage him to put the cups and spoons on the saucers. Have a 'tea party' with him and one of his dolls,

— Give him a pile of small cars, farm animals, buttons, pegs, spoons and get him to find all the cars, animals etc.

— Make a posting box with a circle and a square cut into the top (a plastic ice-cream container will do) and give him round and square shapes to post. Later on you could add triangles and rectangles.

☐ 'I know where this goes.' Seeing how things fit together and putting pieces together to make simple constructions are important skills – and fun to learn.

— Let him build towers of 2 or 3 blocks and then higher towers.

— Give him practice with simple puzzles.

— Give him a short length of curtain wire and some big bright beads with large holes to thread on the wire.

— Collect small pictures of familiar things and paste small groups of them into a scrapbook with his help.

— Encourage him to 'draw' with a water-based felt-tip pen, a ball-point pen or a good wax crayon. Show him how to hold it about half way down with his index finger and thumb on opposite sides.

☐ 'This is what makes it go.' Your child eventually learns that some objects have to be operated in special ways before they will work. Some things to think of in this area:

— Does he understand how to use a wall switch to turn a light on and off?

— Give him a felt-tip pen with the top on and see if he knows he has to take it off before he can write with the pen.

Concepts and Rules are Learned

Your child will enjoy handling more difficult play equipment if you allow him to experiment. He does not always have to do it the correct way, but can try out different solutions, gradually realising which is 'right' and which is 'wrong'. He will see that some shapes are alike, some different, as with colours and sizes. He is beginning to learn some *concepts and rules* about things which are the basics of skills like weighing, measuring, putting things in order, knowing where things belong. A father of a Down's Syndrome boy gave us some good advice on teaching children at this stage: 'What you try and do is help them the best way you can without doing it. It's so easy to say 'Right, I'll show you how to do it' You've got to give them a chance to work things out for themselves.'

The Sixth Step (Developmental Level 2½ – 4 years)

Your Child Still Needs Your Help

By now, your child may well be at a preschool, a special school, or receiving help but, hopefully, you will still be very involved in his learning, and able to provide many opportunities for thinking and coping around the home. If your child has reached this developmental level, he will now have a good range of manipulative skills and a fair understanding of language, allowing him to both comprehend and be active in his world. Concept learning continues to develop during this stage and this helps your child to see relationships between things, to sort out his world and know what goes with what, and where they belong. Thus, he feels much more confident and sure of his ability to cope. The thinking skills we can encourage now are:

Help Your Child learn Relationships

analysis – taking things apart to see how they are made.
synthesis – putting things together to see how they fit.
seriation – putting things in order.
classification – putting things that belong together in groups.

A father of a Down's Syndrome girl seemed to know a lot about teaching his child about relationships when he told us about a particular task: 'I tried to teach her three things: I tried to teach her which is a circle and which is a square, the difference between red and yellow, and which was the big one and which was the little one. So I told her to pick up the big yellow one and she did.'

Ways in which you can help your child to develop an understanding of relationships are listed below:

☐ Provide simple take-apart toys, snap-beads, and jigsaws.

☐ Collect broken objects such as a cup with the handle broken off, a doll with a head or arm off, a shoe with the buckle off or the lace out, a clock with a number or a hand missing, a teapot without a spout. Give one or two to your child, with the broken-off piece, and help him find the right place to 'mend' the object. In the same way, help him pin the tail on to a drawing of a donkey. Also the ears, nose, eyes, a leg and a hoof. He could also replace features on a drawing of a child.

☐ Cut out large pictures of children, toys or animals from magazines and stick them on to cardboard. Then cut each picture into two or three pieces and help the child put them together.

☐ Show him how to thread cotton reels on to thin cord or wire, to make bracelets or necklaces. Make 'jewellery' out of paperchains.

☐ Give him a doll with some easily removable clothes, and a shoe box for a bed, with some bedclothes. Provide a doll's tea set or some unbreakable life-size tea things.

☐ After visits to interesting places, use his toys, blocks, etc., to build a replica and talk about where the different things go, for example, a farm – the sheep in the paddock, pigs in the pen, cows in the shed, car and tractor in the garage.

☐ Collect a few things from three or four rooms in the house. Put them into groups – all the kitchen things, all the bathroom things, etc.

☐ Sort his animals out into groups of sheep, cows, horses, etc.

☐ Group his vehicles into cars, trucks, vans, etc.

☐ Provide a pile of buttons and sort them into groups of colours or sizes.

☐ Let him learn to lay the table and sort out the cutlery drawer.

☐ Cut a piece of dowelling into different lengths and get him to put them in order from the shortest to the longest.

☐ Collect some empty tins of different sizes, clean them and make sure they are safe and then put them in order from the smallest to largest.

Given these ideas as a basis, think of other ways of collecting similar material from the garden, beach or countryside. Let your child try out various ways of sorting, arranging, and putting them together. Encourage him to tell you about why he chooses to try each different way. You might also like to borrow or buy a wooden construction set or plastic building blocks and encourage him to begin putting the pieces together. They need not 'be' anything, but encourage him to tell you about them if he wants to.

Your child now has the use of many important thinking skills. He can cope with the world at his level pretty well. Now he is ready to look to the future. We hope that your awareness of the great achievements he has made, and your own vital contribution to them, will be reward enough for your time and patience.

Remember:

- [ ] *You can help your child learn how to think.*
- [ ] *Your child learns to think through play.*
- [ ] *Everyday objects and experiences are important.*
- [ ] *Attention to tasks is an important skill for your child to learn.*
- [ ] *Children go through different stages in the way they think.*

Elizabeth Straton

8 Independence in Toileting, Dressing and Grooming

I'd put her pants on her . . . You would put one leg through and then fit the other one through and she would take the other one off. Everything is so slow, sort of hard. Even getting her arms in the right position, you don't know whether you have a joint out of place or it is just her resisting you. I have found lately that she is getting harder and harder to dress.

Mother of severely handicapped girl

Being able to take care of ourselves is something we all take for granted. We've dressed and undressed ourselves so often that we don't even have to think about how we do it any more. It's the same with going to the toilet, or washing, or brushing our teeth. The many little actions that go together to allow us to perform a given task effectively are often unnoticed when we become good at doing it.

Have you ever thought about the many little steps which you have learnt in order to complete a task? Next time you brush your teeth, try to observe what you do. Start from the moment you pick up your toothbrush, and finish when you put it back to where you got it. Try to work out which skills you have used in each step of the process – for example, the skills involved in unscrewing the top of the tube and squeezing out just a little toothpaste on to the brush.

Being able to take care of yourself isn't something which 'just happens'. As with any skill, it must be learned.

The major self-help skills every child must learn and which

we discuss in this chapter are:
- ☐ dressing and undressing
- ☐ toileting
- ☐ personal cleanliness and grooming.

Independence is Important for Everybody

All children need to learn to take care of themselves. If your child can't manage to get her pants down by herself, she can't go to the toilet unaided. If your child always needs help with dressing, she has to rely on someone else to get her ready in the morning, to change dirty clothes, and to get her ready for bed at night.

Some children will always be restricted to some degree by the very nature of their handicap, but still it is important to look for ways in which they can be encouraged to become increasingly self reliant. Independence has advantages for all concerned.

First, success breeds success. The thrill of being able to do things for herself, along with praise from others for these successes, increases your child's self confidence and encourages her to do more. The more competent she gets, the more confident she feels about herself and her abilities.

Second, as your child learns to do more for herself, you will have more time for other activities, including more time to spend with her in other interesting ways.

Third, the more independent she is, the less obvious her handicap, both to herself and to others.

DRESSING

If we look at what we call 'dressing', we see that there are two major areas. The first skills, which are easier for children to learn, are those of getting clothing off and on. Different garments require different skills. The second set of skills involves control of hands and fingers and leads to unfastening and fastening of clothing once it is on.

Start by Finding out What Your Child Can Do

1. It is very important that you first find out what she is able to do now. Look very carefully at the chart and tick what she can do *by herself* now.

	Dressing			Fastening	
	Takes off	Puts on		Undoes	Does up
Socks			Velcro		
Vest			Press Studs		
T-shirt			Zips		
Pants			Buttons		
Shoes			Buckles		
Skirt			Ties		
Jersey			Laces		
Shirt/blouse					
Cardigan					
Dress					
Coat					

Work Steps out for Your Child

2. Work out where she is having difficulty. For example:
    ☐ Can she grasp her pants?
    ☐ Can she bend forward while standing and not fall over?
    ☐ Can she stand on one foot?

Make the Steps Small

3. Most skills to be learned should be broken down into a series of very small steps. Go through the task yourself and write down each step, so you know exactly *what* it involves. Watch how other people do the task. This will show you what to teach and *how* to teach it.

Increase Self Help by Reducing Assistance

4. When teaching these steps, your child may need some

help. Give it to her by placing your hands over hers, and guiding her movements. As she gets better at that step, gradually help her less – lighten your touch. Don't help her once, then suddenly take your hands away, and expect her to do it. Each of the steps will take her a little time. If she gets stuck, your steps may be too big for her. Don't try to move ahead too quickly, but work at *her* pace.

Go on to the next step when she can repeat the action consistently *by herself*.

Reward Successes

5.   When teaching skills to your child, it is very important to reward each of her successes, no matter how small, *at once*, as we have discussed in chapter 4. Don't forget to tell her exactly how pleased you are with each try she makes. As she improves, you can expect a little more from her each time before you reward her.

Teach by Backward Chaining

6.   A technique which is often successful in teaching skills to children is one known as *backward chaining*. This means that you use small steps and you work from the

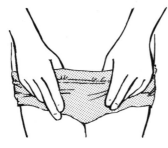

Figure 13 Taking her pants off
What she needs:
1. grasp
2. balance
3. pants with loose waist band.

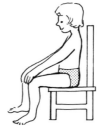

What you need:
1. a chair, right size for child
2. little rewards, e.g. raisins.

end of a task back towards the beginning. In other words, you teach the last step first, the second-to-last step next, and so on.

The following is an example of a way you could teach your child one of the undressing skills using this technique. (If you find some of these steps are too big for your child, break them down into still smaller tasks).

P = Parent (What *you* do)

C = Child (What *she* does)

Your child should be wearing underpants, panties, or elastic-waisted shorts.

1. P – Take her pants down, so that one foot is left inside the pants leg.
     – Sit her on a chair which is her size (make sure she can sit with her feet flat on the floor).
     – Say 'Take your pants off'.
   C – *She bends forward from the waist.*
     – *She grasps her pants with both hands, with her fingers on the outside and her thumbs tucked inside.*
     – *She lifts her foot off the floor and pushes the pants off.*
   P – Reward and praise her for taking them off.

2. P – As for Step 1, but this time leave both of her feet inside the pants legs.
   C – *She first lifts one foot and pushes the pants off it, then lifts her other foot and pushes the pants right off.*
   P – Reward and praise her for taking them off.

3. P – Start with her standing with her pants at her knees.
   C – *She bends over and grasps her pants, pushes them down to her ankles, then sits down on the chair and repeats Step 2.*
   P – Reward and praise her for taking them off.

4. P – As for Step 3, but with her pants at hip level.
   C – *While she is standing with her pants at hip level, get her to push them down and then sit her down on the chair and repeat Step 2.*
   P – Reward and praise her for taking them off.

5. P – As for Step 4, but with her pants at waist level.
       Make sure that her thumbs are tucked inside the
       waist of her pants and her fingers grasp the outside,
       just by the hip.

    C – *She bends over and grasps her pants, pushes them*

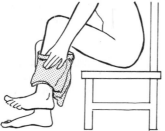

Taking off: Step 1   Taking off: Step 2

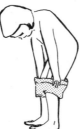
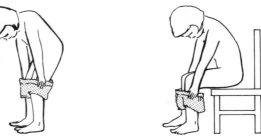

Taking off: Step 3

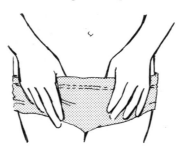

Taking off: Step 4

down to her ankles, then sits on a chair and repeats Step 2.

P – Reward and praise her for taking them off.

6. P – As for Step 5, but this time don't use the chair (for children able to balance).

   C – *She takes her pants off, from her waist, using the grasp described in Step 5, and takes them off over one foot, then the other. To do this, she must balance, first on one foot, then the other. At first she may need some help in balancing (see general hints on dressing given on Page 111).*

   P – Reward and praise her for taking them off.

If you look at putting her pants on, you will find that you can follow the undressing steps in reverse:

1. Start with her pants at hip level and get her to pull them up to her waist,

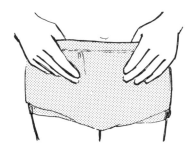

Taking off: Step 5

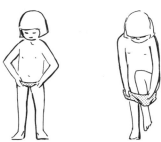

Taking off: Step 6

2. then go from hips to waist,
3. from knees to waist,
4. up from both ankles,
5. over one ankle with the other foot free,
6. then get her to put the pants legs over each of her feet in turn, and pull them up,
7. and finally, get her to pick up her pants, gathering the material, and holding them ready to put over her feet.

What are Some First Steps with Other Clothing?

Using the same step-by-step system, the first step in:
☐ taking off a T-shirt is
— to raise her hands and pull the neck band off the top of her head.
☐ putting on a T-shirt is
— to pull it from chest to waist level.

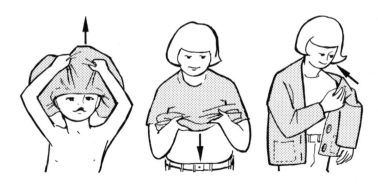

Figure 14

☐ putting on a coat is
   — to pull the coat up over one shoulder, with the hand
   that is already in a sleeve.
☐ buttoning is
   — to slide the last piece of button through the edge of
   the buttonhole.

The following is a way of using the backward chaining
method to teach your child to unzip and to zip up.

Before you start teaching your child, watch for her to
have developed sufficient strength in her hands to successfully grasp both her jacket and the zipper tab.

P = Parent (What you do).
C = Child (What she does).

Unzipping

1. P – Unzip your child's jacket, but leave the last step
       (lifting the tab out of the slot). Say "Lift it out". If
       she has trouble, stand behind her, and use your
       hands over hers to lift the tab out of the slot.
       Gradually lessen your assistance, until she is doing
       it by herself.
   C – *Grasps jacket in either hand and lifts tab out of
       slot.*
   P – Reward and praise her for lifting the tab out of the
       slot.

2. P – Unzip your child's jacket to a few inches from the
       bottom.
   C – *Holds jacket in one hand. Holds zipper tab with
       other hand, slides down to bottom, and lifts tab out
       of the slot.*
   P – Reward and praise her.

3. P – Unzip your child's jacket to half-way.
   C – *Repeats as in Step 2.*
   P – Reward and praise her.

4. P – Ask your child to unzip her jacket.
   C – *Unzips her jacket from the top, and lifts the tab
       from the slot.*
   P – Reward and praise her.

Zipping

1. P – Zip your child's jacket nearly to the top.
    C – *Holds jacket firmly with one hand. Zips from three-quarters to top.*
    P – Reward and praise her for zipping up her jacket.
2. P – Zip your child's jacket to half-way.
    C – *Holds jacket firmly with one hand. Zips from half-way to top.*
    P – Reward and praise her for zipping up her jacket.
3. P – Zip your child's jacket a quarter of the way up.
    C – *Holds jacket firmly with one hand. Zips from a quarter way up to the top.*
    P – Reward and praise her for zipping up her jacket.

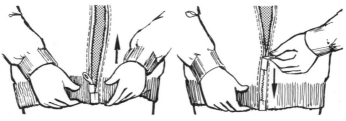

1. Lift tab out of slot.   *2. Unzip and lift tab out of slot.*

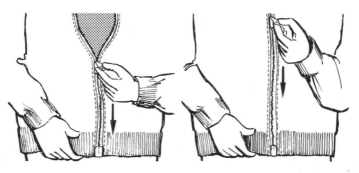

3. Unzip from halfway and lift tab out of slot.   *4. Unzip from top and lift tab out of slot.*

Figure 15   Unzipping.

4. P – Ask your child to zip her jacket up. Help her at first
           by standing behind her, using your hands over hers
           to slide the tab in. As she gets better at it, gradually
           lessen your assistance.
     C – *Slides tab in, and zips jacket up.*
     P – Reward and praise her for zipping up her jacket.

General Hints on Dressing

1. Choose a time when neither of you is in a hurry. Not
    allowing enough time will probably mean you do too
    much for her. Be patient and help her to help herself.
2. Make dressing a pleasurable experience. Start from
    when she's very young, and make dressing a time when

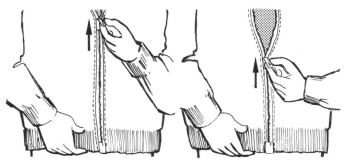

1. Zip from threequarters up to   2. Zip from halfway to top.
top.

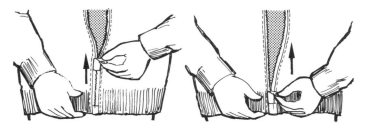

3. Zip from quarter up to top.   4. Place tab in slot and zip up.
                                  Figure 16 Zipping.

you play peek-a-boo and have fun together. As soon as she is able, dress her sitting or standing (with support if needed) so she can see what is happening. Let her try dressing and undressing you or another child.

3. Make sure her clothes fit, but that they also have 'give' and are not too tight for her to manage.

4. A clear marking of a coloured iron-on-patch, e.g. an animal patch inside the back of garments, will show her which way round the garment goes on. It will also help her to identify her clothes.

5. Keep the same articles of clothing in the same place – so she learns her pants are in one drawer, T-shirts in the next drawer. Keep articles which go on together in the same place, e.g., vests and underpants, T-shirts and shorts.

6. Lay her clothes out for her in the right order for putting them on.

7. When taking her pants off, if balance is difficult, let her kneel, lean against a wall, or lean in a corner.

8. The following suggestions might make learning dressing and fastening a little easier for your child:

   ☐ boxer shorts instead of pants with a zip and buckle
   ☐ velcro instead of buttons and zips
   ☐ front fastenings on dresses
   ☐ a key-ring attached to a zip tab
   ☐ plain socks instead of patterned (it doesn't matter if one is on inside out), non-clinging stretch-type socks
   ☐ buttons sewn on with shirring elastic
   ☐ a loop of elastic to fit around the button, instead of a button-hole
   ☐ buttoning, stud or zip pockets with a surprise inside
   ☐ large buttons instead of small ones
   ☐ vertical button-holes before horizontal ones
   ☐ button-holes which aren't too tight or too loose
   ☐ raglan sleeves and loose necks
   ☐ a coloured patch on arm and sleeve to identify which arm goes into which sleeve.

For specific help with physically handicapped children, ask your family doctor for a referral to the occupational therapy department of your nearest hospital. There are many tips which they can give you designed especially to help your child.

TOILET-TRAINING

Toilet-training is also a skill which may be broken down into a number of small steps. Before you start toilet-training your child, remember:
☐ Learning bladder and bowel control varies considerably for each child. All toilet-training is dependent upon your child's having reached a certain level of physical maturity. The muscles which help a child to "hold on" generally function properly only after she has learned to walk. Training, therefore, should be started *only* when your child shows you she is ready.
☐ Don't let *her* train *you* to catch her!
☐ Training should be calm, consistent and without fuss.

Find Out What Your Child Can Do

Tick off on the toileting chart what your child can do:
    Lets you know when wet or dirty ☐
    Shows some regularity of bladder and bowel motions ☐
    Uses potty/toilet when placed on it ☐
    Indicates need to go to toilet ☐
    Toilet-trained with occasional 'accidents' ☐
    Uses toilet for bowel movements ☐
    Supervised toileting during the day ☐
    Independent in toileting during the day ☐
    Has bladder and bowel control at night ☐
Over a period of at least 5 days, check your child every 10 minutes for one hour. Do this three times each day and write

down the result. You may get a chart which looks something like this:

9.00 – *Dry*
9.10 – *Wet*
9.20 – *Dry*
9.30 – *Dry*
9.40 – *Dry*
9.50 – *Dry*
10.00 – *Wet and bowel motion*

Keep the chart handy so you can easily write down what happens.

Work Steps out for Your Child

When you have kept this record for 5 days, look at what has happened and see if your child has established a regular pattern. For example, she may wet approximately every hour to hour and a half, or she may always have a bowel motion around 10 o'clock each day.

If you don't get a pattern of the same thing occurring around the same time, your child may not be ready to start toilet-training yet.

If some regularity is obviously established, you can make a toileting schedule which will tally with the times when she usually wets. This means that you place her on the potty at the times when it is most likely that she will use it. Don't forget to reward her and to tell her how pleased you are with what she has done, every time she uses the potty.

General Hints on Toileting

1. Train bladder control before bowel control.
2. If she has an accident, change her without fuss or attention.
3. Give her plenty of liquids. This means it will be more likely that she will use the potty while she is sitting on it.
4. Keep your child's potty in the toilet so she comes to associate it with going to the toilet. Make sure that

what she's using is comfortable for her, whether it's a potty-chair or a child's toilet seat. Try a box or footstool to help her to reach the toilet seat and for her to rest her feet on.

5. Don't leave her sitting on the toilet or potty by herself, and don't keep her sitting for prolonged periods. If she hasn't used the toilet in 5 or 10 minutes, take her off, without fuss. Don't frighten her by flushing the toilet whilst she's sitting on it. Let her flush it with you after she has pulled up her pants.

6. Give her a familiar toy to hold whilst she is sitting. Don't give her new or noisy toys which will distract her.

7. Make meal-times regular and watch her diet so you don't need to use laxatives.

8. Keep her clothing simple, so that she can get her pants up and down easily. Put her into training pants when you want to start training her.

9. If she starts to have an accident, don't fuss. Take her to the toilet, quickly but calmly. Even when she is trained she may have an occasional accident. Deal with these without fuss.

10. If you have difficulty in establishing toilet-training with your child, get your family doctor or paediatrician to check that there isn't a physical cause.

WASHING AND GROOMING

Your child will find it much easier to learn to wash and groom herself if her training follows a regular schedule. Teach her, for instance, to wash her hands before every meal, and each time she goes to the toilet. In this way you'll help her to learn which acts follow each other during the day.

Tick off on the chart what your child can do.

Find Out What Your Child Can Do
Helps with washing hands   ☐

Helps with washing face ☐
Helps whilst being bathed ☐
Washes hands ☐
Washes face ☐
Dries hands ☐
Dries face ☐
Washes and dries face and hands ☐
Bathes self with supervision ☐
Brushes teeth ☐
Brushes hair ☐
Combs hair ☐
Blows nose ☐

Increase Self-help by Reducing Assistance

At first, when she is learning many of these skills, she may need your help. Put your hands over hers for guidance, then gradually lighten your touch.

Here is a way you can teach her how to wash her hands:
Try following these seven steps. Remember that you and your child are working backwards, and so her first task is what you normally would do *last*. When she can do that step successfully then move to the next step. At Step 2 for example, you and she will be carrying out the whole sequence together, until the last two steps, and what you would be expecting her to do is to put her hands in the water, rinse them, and to pull out the plug. At the end of each new step, ask her to perform the tasks set for the steps that have already been taught. Praise her for performing these correctly.

P = Parent (What *you* do).
C = Child (What *she* does).

Your child should be standing at the right height to comfortably reach the basin and the basin should have warm water in it for each step.

1. P – Tell her to pull out the plug. Help her to do it if necessary. Make sure the plug is loose.
    C – *She grasps the plug chain and pulls.*
    P – Reward and praise her for pulling out the plug.

2. Refill the basin with warm water. Soap her hands.
   - P – Tell her to put her hands in the water and rinse them. Show her what to do.
   - C – *She puts her hands in the water and rinses them until all the soap is off.*
   - P – Reward and praise her for rinsing her hands. Tell her to pull the plug.
3. P – Tell her to rub her hands together, both the front and the back, and separating her fingers. Show her what to do.
   - C – *She washes her hands all over.*
   - P – Reward and praise her for washing her hands.
4. P – When she has soap all over her hands, ask her to put the soap back.
   - C – *She puts the soap back.*
   - P – Reward and praise her for putting the soap back.
5. P – Give her the soap and get her to rub it over the hands.
   - C – *She rubs the soap over her hands.*
   - P – Reward and praise her for rubbing the soap over her hands.
6. P – Ask her to put her hands and the soap in the water.
   - C – *She wets her hands and the soap.*
   - P – Reward and praise her for wetting her hands and the soap.
7. P – Ask her to pick up the soap.
   - C – *She picks up the soap and holds it.*
   - P – Reward and praise her for picking up the soap.

When your child can wash her hands by herself, teach her to fill the basin. The steps for learning this would go like this:

1. turning the tap off
2. checking the water-level (a mark on the side of the basin may help her to know when the basin is full enough)
3. checking the water-temperature
4. putting the plug in
5. turning the taps on, (teach how to turn the cold tap on first and off last).

Make sure she can reach hand basin easily

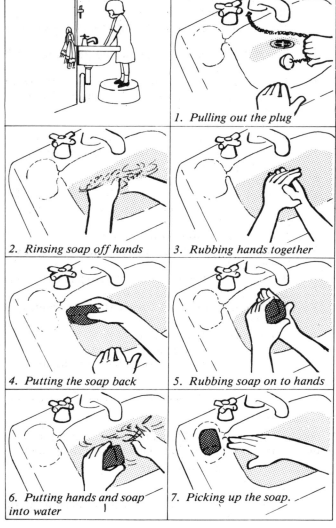

Figure 18   Washing hands.

General Hints on Washing and Grooming

1. When helping your child to learn to wash herself, you should:

   ☐ Turn the hot-water thermostat down so she will not scald herself.

   ☐ Teach her hot and cold – make sure that she knows which tap is which. (Mark the hot tap with red tape where she can easily see it and teach her why it is there.)

   ☐ Keep the soap, facecloth, her toothbrush etc. within easy reach for her and in the same place. Use a small stool or box so that she can reach the basin, and can see into the mirror.

2. When helping your child to brush her teeth, you should:

   ☐ Ask for advice from your dentist.

   ☐ Teach her that the best brush movements are up and down or rotary, rather than sideways.

   ☐ Have a big bathroom mirror so that she can watch herself and her parents cleaning their teeth.

   ☐ Play games together with your toothbrushes.

   ☐ Let her taste the toothpaste, and

   ☐ Don't get one which has too sharp a taste.

   ☐ Don't force the toothbrush into her mouth, or make her keep her mouth open for too long.

   ☐ Use a toothbrush which is the right size for her.

   ☐ Give her a small plastic mug to use in rinsing.

   ☐ Make sure she can hold and drink from the mug, and will spit the water out into the basin, not drink it. (Teach her this by letting her watch you.)

   ☐ Let her practise screwing and unscrewing the tops of empty tubes of toothpaste.

   ☐ Let her practise using two hands together to do

something, e.g. holding a container with one hand whilst taking the lid on and off with the other hand. This will help her with handling the toothbrush and toothpaste tube together.

☐ A small tube of toothpaste is easier to squeeze than a large one (and also more economical if it gets squeezed in the wrong place!).

☐ Teach her to squeeze from a place on the toothpaste tube where she can control the amount coming out. It may help to squeeze a little toothpaste out first so the toothpaste doesn't shoot everywhere.

☐ Match the amount of toothpaste with the head of the brush.

☐ Teach her to break off the toothpaste with a twist.

3. When helping your child to take care of her hair, you should:

☐ Make sure the bristles of the brush aren't too sharp.

☐ Encourage her to turn her hand correctly (again you may need to help her with your hand over hers), both for combing and brushing.

☐ Give her time to play in front of the mirror with toys, so she gets to know what happens when she moves them a certain way, (looking in a mirror and trying to do something is often confusing). Let her also play with her brush and comb in front of the mirror.

☐ Use a comb which suits her and which she finds easy to handle. Some children may prefer a tail-comb.

☐ Let her comb and brush your hair to help practise handling the brush and comb.

Remember to:

☐ *Look at* what *your child is doing and* how *she is doing it.*

☐ *Break tasks down into small steps.*

☐ *Decide* what *you are going to teach and* how *you are going to teach it.*

☐ *Make the steps appropriate for your child.*

☐ *Reward successes.*
Through learning together, both you and your child will gain independence.

Robyn Ward
Barry Parsonson

9 Behaviour Problems can be Managed

I found it very hard to cope with Arnie, day in and day out with things like tantrums . . . . I really could have hurt her, I think.

Mother of deaf girl

She virtually rules the house. We understand that and we can accept it. But it would be nice to have a break.

Father of severely handicapped girl

This chapter looks briefly at three areas of behaviour that sometimes become difficult to manage if not handled carefully. Some parents report that they have 'tried everything' and have still not managed to deal with some behaviour problem. The suggestions offered earlier in chapter 4 and in this chapter require consistent and careful application over a period of time. We don't claim that they work for everyone or with all problems, but they have been found effective in many instances. When trying to manage serious or long-term problem behaviour, it probably is best to seek assistance from psychologists trained in designing and managing treatment programmes. Below are some suggestions for you to consider when wondering how to handle common problem behaviour.

WHINING, TANTRUMS, BREATH-HOLDING AND HEAD-BANGING

Most young children try to get their own way by such

behaviour at some stage. Whether they do so frequently can very much depend on how you react.

Don't give out 'Goodies' for the Sake of Peace

For example, if you are talking on the phone and your child begins to tug at your arm and whine and nag for a biscuit, you may feel tempted to give in for the sake of peace. You may get peace, but only for the moment. He will have learned from his success the first time that nagging and whining when you are on the phone is a good way of getting what he wants, and will probably do it again.

If you don't want to reinforce his behaviour, your best move is to ignore him. If circumstances make this difficult, try asking your caller to wait and get your child started on some activity in a spot where he can see you.

Praise his Good Behaviour

Nod and smile at him while you finish your phone call, if he is playing happily. When you hang up, praise him for being good while you were busy, and spend a little time with him.

Children Work Out when They can get Attention

Children soon learn when you are most likely to get flustered or easily embarrassed by a display of temper, head-banging or breath-holding, and these are the very times when they are likely to make a scene – when you are trying to hold a telephone conversation, making a meal, entertaining visitors, or in a public place. Do your best not to show concern – and don't give way to his demands, or you will increase the likelihood of a repeat performance.

Ignoring takes Effort. Keep at it

It's not easy to ignore a child who seems bent on self-destruction or showing you up in the worst possible situation. If you manage to ignore him the first time, his reaction will be to try to make his behaviour even more noticeable – to whine louder, to stamp and yell more fiercely, to hold his breath all over the place, or to bang his head harder and more often.

You may then fear that ignoring him has only made things worse, and decide to give in. But this phase is a sign that ignoring him is beginning to work, and if you can keep it up, his outbursts should lessen, and eventually die away altogether.

If you do give way at this stage, you will have taught him that he didn't make a big enough fuss the first time, and the worse his behaviour, the more chance he has of getting your attention.

It's worth remembering that tantrums pass, at worst breath-holding will end in a brief harmless faint, and head-banging gets painful!

If you find that you simply cannot ignore his behaviour, you could try the Time-Out procedure (described in chapter 4) as an alternative.

BEDTIME AND SLEEPING PROBLEMS

Parents often look forward to getting their children off to bed so that they can settle down for a chat, to read, or to watch TV. Interruptions such as calls from the bedroom for drinks of water, or from someone toddling out saying they would rather watch TV than sleep, can be annoying.

Make Bedtime a Nice Time

Sometimes this kind of behaviour becomes part of the regular bedtime routine. When this happens, take a look at the way you organise getting him off to bed. Try to make it a pleasant process that starts before he gets overtired. Try praising him for bedtime activities like brushing his teeth, going to the toilet, and getting into his pyjamas. Once he's in bed, be sure he has all of his 'essential' things like his cuddly toy and a small drink of water on his bedside table. Sit or lie beside him and have a chat about the good things that happened today or special events coming up soon. Read him a brief story. Before you leave, ask him if there is anything he wants, settle him down, and say goodnight (and mean it!). If he doesn't like the dark, try leaving the passage light on and his door open, or buy a night-light. Leave him to go to sleep.

Don't Answer Unnecessary Calls or Cries

If he calls for you or cries, judge the importance of the matter. If possible, ignore him. If you *must* go to him, check that there is nothing else before you leave him again. Ignore any more calls.

If he comes out, calmly but firmly take him back to bed, tuck him in, and tell him to go to sleep. Of he is persistent at getting up and wanting to play or watch TV, shut the door between his bedroom and the lounge. Let him cry in the passage if he must, let him go to sleep there, but don't let him come out and join you.

He Should Sleep in his Own Bed

Some children wake up at night and demand attention. A night-light can help if he is scared when he wakes in the dark. It can allow him to find his drink of water or the way to the toilet. You will encourage your child to get up if you play with him or take him into your own bed. If he tries to join you in bed, take him back to his own bed and settle him in with as little fuss and attention as possible. If he keeps trying, let him go to sleep on the floor or outside your bedroom door. If he tantrums or screams, don't give in. Letting him sleep with you on a regular basis can make your life very difficult.

Look at Your Child's Sleeping Pattern

If you have a child who does not sleep well at night, and there is no medical reason, look at his sleeping pattern. Maybe his afternoon rest is making up for sleep lost at night, or perhaps some bedtime activity excites him too much. Does he have too many or too few bedclothes? Think about what you do when he wakes up at night. Try some different approaches to the problem. Ignore him. In time he will get tired and sleep. It may take a week or so of rough nights with no daytime rests for him. Be sure to work out how to get some sleep yourself. Try a system of praise for each 'peaceful' night, with a special reward for three in a row, then, later, for a whole week, ten days, then for a fortnight in a row, etc. Try to get a new sleep pattern established.

GETTING ALONG WITH OTHER CHILDREN

Children with special needs sometimes have difficulty in mixing with other children, both within (siblings) and outside (peers) the family. Problems with siblings come from at least two sources:

Share Your Time with All of the Family

First, as parents you may find a lot of time is taken up attending to the special needs of your child and you may expect your other children to manage more or less for themselves. They may discover that you give them more attention when they are unco-operative or misbehave, or when they tease or exclude the handicapped child. You may think they are jealous and try to explain to them why you have to devote extra time to one family member. However, you should take a look at your commitments to your family, perhaps planning to divide your attention more evenly, to praise and reward the other children when they do the chores or join in activities with their 'special' sibling. Consider giving them their own particular time when they are the centre of attention.

Second, the nature of some handicaps is such that your child may be limited in the variety and types of interaction he can have with other children. He may have difficulty understanding 'rules', he may find it hard to communicate, or he may tire quickly. Such restrictions may mean that he gets left out completely, or that he gets irritable, refuses to co-operate, or has tantrums – perhaps because he can never win, or as a way to get the other children to fit in with his wishes.

Invent Games that are Fun for All

When this happens you could encourage the other children to adapt games so that he can join in more easily, or to invent new games that all can play. You can then praise them all for co-operative play and good relationships instead of only giving attention to squabbles or teasing. Also, children with special needs should be taught how to relate to other children in appropriate ways.

Help Children Get on Together

Interactions with peers may be more of a problem because children from outside of the family can be less understanding. They may taunt, tease, or make fun of a child who is 'different'. Much of this may stem from ignorance, especially as the integration of children with special needs into the various levels of the educational system is not as widespread as might be wished.

Your natural urge to protect your child from unsympathetic non-handicapped children does not help. You can't isolate your child from all of the unpleasant aspects of the real world. Instead, try to teach both your child and his peers to get along together and to learn that everyone has a place and a contribution to make. This is best done by encouraging co-operation, praising behaviour you like to see, and by your own example.

Remember to

☐ *pay attention to 'good' behaviour*
☐ *ignore 'bad' behaviour: it usually works – if you keep at it*
☐ *be consistent*
☐ *share your time with all the family*
☐ *teach children to get on together.*

Barry Parsonson

10 Some Key Services

If you have a child with special needs, you can obtain assistance from a variety of state and voluntary services. While some are readily available only in larger towns and cities, even if you live in the country you will have access to practical assistance and advice. Since it is beyond the scope of this book to give a complete listing of all the services, groups and organisations which are available we have concentrated on the main ones. Also, rather than attempting to list all the local branches of the various societies, we have given the addresses, where applicable, of the head offices.

HELP FROM THE STATE

Department of Health and Social Security
You should be able to get help initially from your own doctor and health visitor. Your doctor can refer you to specialists on the National Health and your health visitor has, or can obtain, leaflets dealing with special problems you may face over day to day matters such as feeding. If your child is attending a paediatric clinic at a hospital you can also get help there, especially in the form of physiotherapy, speech therapy, occupational therapy.

Don't forget, that as the parent of a handicapped child, you are eligible for a variety of allowances, apart from the basic family allowance. For example, there is the Attendance Allowance for children over 2 who need a great deal of care day and night; the Mobility Allowance for children over 5 who are virtually unable to walk; Supplementary

Benefit for handicapped children on special diets, etc. You can get details of these and other benefits from your local Social Security office. There is also a Family Fund, Beverly House, Shipton Road, York., which awards discretionary lump sums for special needs such as help with transport, holidays, laundry.

Under the Chronically Sick and Disabled Persons Act local councils can give grants and help to the handicapped through the Social Services Department. Among the services available are home helps, travelling arrangements or a petrol allowance if you yourself have to transport your child to and from a special school or hospital. Cuts in local authority spending have made it harder to get help but it is always worth asking.

Department of Education and Science
All children have a right to an education – and a handicapped child is no exception. Your Local Education Authority has a duty to provide a suitable school place for your child although, in very exceptional cases, individual teaching can be arranged. To find out more contact your local education officer in charge of special education.

Schools run by LEA's are listed in the Education Year Book, Longmans and you can look at a copy of this in your local library. Maybe there is not a suitable school for your child in your area, in which case the above book also lists independent and non-maintained schools which may fit the bill. If your child has to go to one of these schools, or to a school run by another LEA, most LEA's will agree to sponsor her.

Various grants and concessions are also available. To find out about them you should contact your local Education Welfare Officer either through the school or your local education office. This officer can also help to arrange sessions with various specialists in the department such as educational psychologists, speech therapists, physiotherapists. She or he may also be able to lend a hand in arranging other matters such as holidays and put you in touch with various holiday play schemes.

For further advice and information you could also contact the National Council for Special Education, Downham School, Horn Lane, Plymstock, Devon, Plymouth 43214.

Voluntary Organisations

Many of the organisations listed here were founded by parents of handicapped children. Although you will be able to get quite a large amount of basic information and help from your family doctor or clinic, these groups are often the best place to turn to, not only for up-to-date information, but also for practical advice on every aspect of your child's handicap from people who have experienced the failures and successes themselves.

The head office of an organisation can usually put you in touch with your nearest local group, where you will have a chance to meet parents with similar problems to your own. The larger societies can also provide a great deal of information in the form of leaflets and their own book lists and they often have their own assessment and treatment centres, schools and trained advisors to help you decide on the best ways to educate your child.

If you have any difficulties in contacting a particular society, since addresses and phone numbers do change, check with the Voluntary Council for Handicapped Children, 8 Wakley Street, London, E.C.1. 01-278 9441. As well as having a very comprehensive information service on sources of help, the council also publishes several fact sheets on aspects of help for various handicaps and a useful free booklet for parents called Help Starts Here.

Voluntary Groups

General

The following organisations can offer basic help and advice both verbally and in the form of leaflets on handicaps in general. Many offer ideas and schemes to help extend the area of your child's activities – playgroups, sports etc.

REFERENCES

Dr. Barnado's, Tanner's Lane, Barkingside, Essex 01-550 8822

British Sports Association for the Disabled, Stoke Mandeville Stadium, Harvey Road, Aylesbury, Bucks. 0296 84848

Disability Alliance, 5 Netherhall Gardens, London, N.W.3. 01 794 1536

Disabled Living Foundation, 346 Kensington High Street, London, W.14. 01-602 2491

Handicapped Adventure Playground Association, Palace Playground, Fulham Palace, Bishop's Avenue, London, S.W.6. 01-736 4443

Invalid Children's Aid Association, 126 Buckingham Palace Road, London, W.1. 01-730 9891

Lady Hoare Trust for Physically Disabled Children, 7 North Street, Midhurst, West Sussex. 073 081 3696

MIND, National Association for Mental Health, 22 Harley Street, London, W.1. 01-637 0741

National Association for Maternal and Child Welfare, 1 South Audley Street, London, W.1. 01-491 2772

National Association of Swimming Clubs for the Handicapped, 4 Hillside Gardens, Northwood, Middx. 09274-27784

National Association for the Welfare of Children in Hospital (NAWCH), 7 Exton Street, London, S.E.1. 01-261 1738

National Campaign for the Young Chronic Sick, 94 Marlborough Flats, Whitton Street, London, S.W.3.

National Children's Bureau, 8 Wakley Street, London, E.C.1. 01-278 9441

National Children's Home, 85 Highbury Park, London, N.1. 01-226 2033

National Council for One-Parent Families, 255 Kentish Town Road, London, N.W.5. 01- 267 1361

National Fund for Research into Crippling Diseases, Vincent House, Springfield Road, Horsham, Sussex.

The Patients Association, 11 Dartmouth Street, London, S.W.1. 01 222 4992

PHAB Clubs (Physically Handicapped and Able-Bodied), 42 Devonshire Street, London, W.1. 01 637 7475

Pre-School Playgroups Association, Alford House, Aveline Street, London, S.E.11 01-582 8871 (Special Needs Advisor: Mrs. Delphine Knight, 10 Woodhaw, Egham, Surrey. 07843 37184)

Riding for the Disabled Association, National Agricultural Centre, Kenilworth, Warwickshire. 0203 56107

Rudolf Steiner Association, Rudolf Steiner House, 35 Park Road, London, N.W.1. 01 723 4400

Specific

Afasic Association (Association for all Speech Impaired Children), 347 Central Market, Smithfield, London, E.C.1. 01 236 3632

Association for Children with Heart Disorders, 536 Colne Road, Reedley, nr. Burnley, Lancs.

Association of Parents of Vaccine Damaged Children, Mrs. Rosemary Fox, 2 Church Street, Shipston-on-Stour, Warwks. 0608 61595

Association for Research into Restricted Growth, 3 West Croft, West End, Clevedon, Avon.

Asthma Research Council, 12 Pembridge Square, London, W.2. 01 229 1149

Breakthrough Trust, 66 Greenwich South Street, London, S.E.10 01 691 6229

British Diabetic Association, 10 Queen Anne Street, London, W.1.

British Dyslexia Association, 4 Hobart Place, London, S.W.1. 01-235 8111

British Epilepsy Association, 3 Alfred Place, London, W.C.1. 01-580 2704

British Heart Foundation, 57 Gloucester Place, London, W.1. 01-935 0185

British Polio Fellowship, Bell Close, West End Road, Ruislip, Middx.

British Retinitis Pigmentosa Society, 24 Palmer Close, Redhill, Surrey. Redhill 61937

British Rheumatism and Arthritis Association, 6 Grosvenor Crescent, London, S.W.1. 01-235 0902

British Thoracic and Tuberculosis Association, 30 Britten Street, London, S.W.3. 01 352 2194

Brittle Bone Society, 63 Byron Crescent, Dundee. 0382 87130

Coeliac Society, P.O. Box 181, London, N.W.2. 01 459 2440

Cystic Fibrosis Research Trust, 5 Blyth Road, Bromley, Kent 01 464 7211

Down's Children's Association, Quinborne Centre, Ridgacre Road, Birmingham 32.

Leukemia Research Fund, 43 Great Ormond Street, London, W.C.1. 01 405 0101

Migraine Trust, 45 Great Ormond Street, London, W.C.1. 01-278 2676

Multiple Sclerosis Society (Crack), 286 Munster Road, London, S.W.6. 01-381 4022

Muscular Dystrophy Group of Great Britain, Natrass House, 35 Macaular Road, London, S.W.4. 01-720 8055

National Association for Gifted Children, 1 South Audley Street, London, W.1. 01-499 1188

National Association for Deaf/Blind and Rubella Handicapped, J. Pryce-Owen, Suffolk House, 10 The Butts, Coventry 0203 23308

National Deaf Children's Society, 45 Hereford Road, London, W.2. 01 229 9272

National Eczema Society, 5 Tavistock Place, London, W.C.1. 01-388 4097

National Society for Autistic Children, Mrs M. Everard, 1a Golders Green Road, London, N.W.11. 01 458 4375

National Society for Brain Damaged Children, 35 Larchmere Drive, Hall Green, Birmingham 28 021 777 4284

National Society for Cancer Relief, Michael Sobell House, 30 Dorset Square, London, N.W.1.

National Society for Phenylketonuria and Allied Disorders, 26 Towngate Grove, Mirfield, West Yorkshire.

Partially Sighted Society, Exhall Grange School, Wheelwright Lane, Coventry. 0203 36420

Royal Association in Aid of the Deaf and Dumb, 7 Armstrong Road, London, W.3. 01-743 6187

Royal National Institute for the Blind, 224 Great Portland Street, London, W.1. 01 388 1266.

Royal National Institute for the Deaf, 105 Gower Street, London, W.C.1. 01 387 8033

The Spastics Society, 12 Park Crescent, London, W.1. 01 636 5020

Spina Bifida and Hydrocephalus Association, Tavistock House, North Tavistock Square, London, W.C.1. 01 388 1382

Spinal Injuries Association, 5 Crowndale Road, London, N.W.1. 01-388 6840

11 Useful Books

There is no shortage of useful books to help you to understand and provide for your child with special needs. The list which follows includes books which are specific to particular handicaps, others which apply to all children with special needs, while others are concerned with all babies and children, whether or not they have special needs.

While not all the books we have listed are readily available in bookshops, you should not have too much difficulty in getting hold of most of them. Many of them can be borrowed from a public library – and if your local library does not have a copy one can probably be loaned from another library for you. Most voluntary societies have libraries containing books dealing with specific handicaps – occasionally these books can be borrowed and you can certainly look at them in the library. These societies also have their own booklists, giving details of books they feel are particularly useful.

If you decide you want to buy books which look like being permanently useful for reference and guidance you can either order through your local bookshop or directly from the publisher.

Beresford, P. and Tuckwell, P.
Schools for All. 1977 MIND and
Campaign for the Mentally Handicapped.
A book which discusses the education of the severely handicapped
and argues convincingly that they
should be integrated into the
normal school system. Gives
examples of where this has
happened and how it has worked.

Brinkworth, R. and Collins, Dr. J.
Improving Babies with Down's
Syndrome. Society for Mentally
Handicapped Children.
A descriptive and factual book. An
excellent one to read when you first
hear the news about your child as it
is full of positive thoughts on what
can be done and where you can go
for help.

Browning, E. "I Can't See What
You're Saying". Paul Elek 1972
A good read. The author has
brought up a child with severe
speech disorders and the book is
full of information and practical
advice.

Caplan, F. The First Twelve
Months of Life. Bantam Books
1973
A thorough and readable outline of
normal development in the first
twelve months. Covers such topics
as feeding, crying, sleeping, toys,
socialisation, language, obedience,
memory, fears and imagination.
Relevant to all parents.

Carr, J. Helping Your Handicapped Child: A Step by Step Guide
to Everyday Problems. Penguin
1980
A sensible and comprehensive
explanation of how to use behaviour modification with your mentally handicapped child.

Clarke, A.D.B. and A.M. Practical
Help for Parents of Retarded
Children. Hull Society for Mentally
Handicapped Children.

Chapman, E.K. Visually Handicapped Children and Young
People. Routledge and Kegan Paul
1978
Deals with the social and emotional
development of blind children from
an educational point of view, and
shows what is available in education in this country.

Collins M & D. Kith and Kids – Self
Help for Families of the Handicapped. Souvenir Press 1976
A very positive and practical book
which discusses how parents of
handicapped children can get
together and form self help groups
for mutual support and help.

Cunningham, C and Jeffree, D.
Barnaby Books. Learning Development Aids

Cunningham, C and Sloper P.
Helping Your Handicapped Baby.
Souvenir Press 1978
A book for parents eager to help
their handicapped babies, this one
is highly recommended for its care,
thoroughness and practicality.

Dale, D.M.C. Deaf Children at
home and at school. University of
London Press 1968
A practical book which contains
helpful advice to the parents of
young deaf children. Gives basic
information about deafness and
emphasises home/school co-
operation and the integration of the
deaf into regular schools.

Finnie, N. Handling the Young
Cerebral Palsied Child at Home.
Heinemann Medical Books 1974
A book written specially for

parents by a physiotherapist. It gives detailed guidance on all aspects of care, including the development of movement, bathing, toileting, dressing, feeding and play.

Fraiberg, S. Insights from the Blind. Souvenir Press 1977
Reports the results of a long and intensive study of a group of blind babies and how they were helped to go through 'normal' developmental stages. Although it includes some technical material it also contains useful practical ideas.

Freeman, P. Understanding the Deaf-Blind Child. Heinemann Health Books
Although written for parents of deaf-blind children, much of the information in this book is of value to parents of children with other handicaps.

Furneaux, B. The Special Child. Pelican
An examination of the types of education available to the child with learning difficulties.

Furneaux, B. and Roberts, B (eds) Autistic Children: Teaching, Community and Research Approaches. Henley and Boston London 1977
A comprehensive study of autism. Its main emphases are on the special needs of autistic kids and everyday aspects of dealing with them.

Gibson, D. Down's Syndrome: The Psychology of Mongolism. Cambridge University Press 1978
A critical overview of the biological and psychological development of Down's Syndrome children.

Hannam, C. Parents and Mentally Handicapped Children. Penguin 1980
Charles Hannam is the father of a Down's Syndrome boy. His book is the result of conversations with other parents of children with a range of intellectual handicap.

Hastings, P. and Hayes, B. Encouraging Language Development. Croom Helm, London 1981
Help and advice for parents and professionals. A sensible book with lots of practical advice, no jargon, plenty of illustrations and a good bibliography.

Hunton, Dr. M. Medical Help for Children with Down's Syndrome. Mark and Moody 1980
The book covers all the medical aspects which can face children with Down's Syndrome.

Jeffree, D., McConkey, R. and Hewson, S. Let Me Play/Let Me Speak. Souvenir Press 1977
These two books for parents provide games and activities to stimulate and develop babies and toddlers and children. Let Me Speak is a book of language promoting games for parents to use with handicapped babies and young children.

Larsen, H. Don't Forget Tom. Adam and Charles Black 1974
A sensitive, beautifully illustrated book on a handicapped child that could help brothers and sisters understand handicaps.

Lear, R. Play Helps: Toys and Activities for Handicapped Children. Heinemann Health Books 1977
An illustrated, carefully planned book of play activities based on sight, hearing and touch for

infants, pre-school and school-age children.

Lorber, J. Your Child with Spina Bifida. Available from the Association for Spina Bifida and Hydrocephalus (See Chapter 10). A most useful guide for parents with clear descriptions of the nature of spina bifida and the ways it can be managed.

Lowenfield, B. Our Blind Children – Growing and Learning with Them. Springfield, Illinois; Charles C. Thomas 1964
Covers the pre-school and school-age child with visual handicaps. Consideration is given to such topics as eating, toileting, dressing, play, mobility and language.

Ludlow, J.R. Down's Syndrome; Let's Be Positive.
Down's Children Association (see Ch. 10)
A fascinating account of a survey conducted in Kent among Down's Syndrome children. Aimed at teachers and social workers but still interesting for parents to read as it includes case histories.

McCormack, M. A Mentally Handicapped Child in the Family Constable

Purser, A. You and Your Handicapped Child. Allen and Unwin 1981
A down to earth book by the mother of a handicapped child about the problems and solutions, successes and failures of bringing her up to womanhood.

Peine, H.A. and Howarth, R. Children and Parents: Everyday Problems of Behaviour. Penguin 1975
A short, but very readable, manual designed to help parents solve ordinary everyday problems they may encounter in their children.

Peterson, P. Sally Can't See. Adam and Charles Black 1976
A useful book for helping family members understand visual handicap.

Rapp, D.J. and Frankland, A.W. Allergies – Questions and Answers. Heinemann Health Books 1976
Very clear explanations of all kinds of allergies but with particular attention given to asthma.

Stone, J. and Taylor, F. Handbook for Parents with a Handicapped Child. Arrow.
A comprehensive guide to all imaginable sources of help available.

Personal Stories

One can often get a great deal of comfort and help by reading personal stories either by handicapped people themselves or by their parents. Here are just a few;

Hunt, N. The World of Nigel Hunt. Darwen Finlayson

Schaefer, N. Does She Know She's There? Harper and Row

Wallace, M and Robson, M. On Giant's Shoulders. Corgi

West, P. Words for a Deaf Daughter. Gollancz

Contributors

David Mitchell, Senior Lecturer in Education, Director of Project PATH, University of Waikato, Hamilton, New Zealand

Peter Hallinan, Lecturer in Special Education, Mitchell College of Advanced Education, Bathurst, NSW, Australia

Christine Hilton, Senior Speech Therapist, Carlson School, Auckland, New Zealand

Mary Lane, Research Assistant in Special Education, Project PATH

Jill Mitchell, Lecturer in Education, Hamilton Teachers College, New Zealand

Barry Parsonson, Senior Lecturer in Psychology, University of Waikato, New Zealand

Elizabeth Straton, Director DAWNSTART Project, Psychological Service, Department of Education, Wellington, New Zealand

David Straton, Lecturer in Psychological Medicine, Wellington Clinical School, Wellington Hospital, New Zealand

Robyn Ward, Speech Therapist, Project PATH

Additional Assistance
Vivienne Webb-Hendy, Martha Parker, Project PATH
Val Brooke-White, Continuing Education Unit, Radio New Zealand

PATH is a research project funded by the Education Department, the Mental Health Foundation, the Lottery Board of Control and the IYC Telethon Trust, and supported by the University of Waikato. Its activities include the surveying of parents of children with special needs, the preparation of materials suitable for parents or professionals working with young handicapped children, and an early intervention programme.

DAWNSTART is a project funded in part by the Education Department, the Wellington Clinical School of Wellington Hospital, and the Mental Health Foundation. Its main concern is with working with infants known or suspected to have a handicap. Like PATH, the focus is on helping parents to become more skilled in helping their children's development.